D1283514

WORKING WITH WEST INDIAN FAMILIES

Working with West Indian Families

Sharon-Ann Gopaul-McNicol, Ph.D.

THE GUILFORD PRESS
New York   London

*T*o Mom and Dad
with tenderness, love, and respect

© The Guilford Press 1993
A Division of Guilford Publications, Inc.
72 Spring Street, New York, NY 10012

Printed in the United States of America

This book is printed on acid-free paper.

Last digit is print number: 9 8 7 6 5 4 3 2 1

Library of Congress Cataloging-in-Publication Data

Gopaul-McNicol, Sharon-Ann.
    Working with West Indian families / Sharon-Ann Gopaul-
McNicol.
      p. cm.
    Includes bibliographical references and index.
    ISBN 0-89862-229-8   ISBN 0-89862-024-4 (pbk.)
    1. Social work with minorities—United States. 2. West Indian
Americans—Services for. 3. West Indians. I. Title.
HV3189.A2G65   1993
362.84'00973—dc20   92-31870
                                                            CIP

Preface

I have lived in the United States since 1978, and in that time I have always been amazed how little is generally known about West Indian people. Although questions such as "Is Trinidad in Jamaica?" or "Which part of Jamaica is Grenada?" are rarely asked today (probably due to the influx of American tourists to the various Caribbean islands), a lack of sensitivity to the cultural diversity of West Indian families nonetheless persists. Some teachers and psychologists still suggest that the same techniques employed in working with black American children can be applied to black West Indian children. I believe this to be a serious error. Discussing this issue is difficult for me, because in my own personal and political life I have consciously avoided making distinctions between black Americans and black West Indian Americans. However, at my agency— Multicultural Educational and Psychological Services, P.C.—I conduct several types of groups to aid immigrant families in their cultural adjustment. Through these individual, group, and family sessions with West Indians, coupled with my experiences as a consulting school psychologist and an assistant professor at St. John's University, I have come to realize that a different approach to tutelage and psychotherapy is needed if West Indian families are to acculturate smoothly in this society.

This book is the outcome of five years of research on West Indian families, based on my own practical, clinical, and supervisory experiences. While there has been a proliferation of literature on the political status of West Indians in the West Indies, there has been little research on educational, and particularly psychological, issues with respect to West Indians in the West Indies, the United States, the

v

United Kingdom, and Canada. It is my hope that this book will be used as a point of reference, a sort of clinical tool, to merge current historical, sociopolitical, cultural, educational, familial, and psychological knowledge about West Indian families.

To gain more than a superficial knowledge and to extricate cultural factors that might be pertinent in understanding West Indian families, I felt that clinical interviews, though necessary, would be an insufficient means of attaining a holistic grasp of the West Indian cultural values and beliefs. Therefore I developed several questionnaires to gain an understanding of the values that are unique to the West Indian culture. The Immigrant Self-Concept Scale (Appendix III) and the Immigrant Attitude Survey (Appendix IV) were distributed to 402 West Indian immigrants—236 in the United States, 89 in the United Kingdom, and 77 in Canada. The West Indian Attitude Survey (Appendix V) was distributed to 390 West Indians currently residing in the West Indies. In addition, 56 West Indian immigrant students in the United States were given the Wechsler Intelligence Scale for Children—Revised, the Bender–Gestalt Visual–Motor Test, the Thematic Apperception Test, the Wide Range Achievement Test—Revised, the Woodcock–Johnson Achievement Test, and the Human Figure Drawing Tests. Furthermore, 81 West Indians were informally interviewed— 40 in the United States, 28 in the West Indies, 8 in the United Kingdom, and 5 in Canada. Teachers and mental health workers made up the majority of participants in the informal interviews. The interviews, each of which lasted approximately an hour, focused on such areas as family, education, work values, race, disciplinary measures used, reasons for migration, problems with acculturation, perspectives on the effectiveness of psychotherapeutic interventions, and interisland differences, all of which are discussed in this book. These questionnaires (though not standardized) provided some rudimentary guidelines for understanding West Indian families. Merely responding to the questions helped many participants examine the thoughts and feelings that form the basis of their attitudes and behaviors. Many participants, after responding to some of the questions, said it was the first time they had ever seriously thought about their biases, inhibitions, and other traditionally held beliefs.

Writing this book proved to be simultaneously gratifying and difficult for me: gratifying because I was able to share years of my work with West Indian families, but difficult because of the magnitude of the project. By no means do I profess to know everything about West Indian families, particularly the interisland cultural nuances. However, undertaking this project, coupled with my early years of growing up in Trinidad and Tobago, certainly helped me to shed some traditional cultural encapsulations and instead incorporate the West Indian world perspective in psychotherapy. I hope that West Indian therapists and those working with West Indian families will continue to conduct and publish research, so that we can increase our database and knowledge about West Indian families. The history of West Indians, including their immigration patterns and contributions to the United States, the United Kingdom, and Canada, ought to be studied in greater detail. That, however, is beyond the scope of this book. The main purpose of this book is to increase our psychological, sociopolitical, and educational understanding of West Indian Americans and West Indians in the West Indies. However, in Chapters 9 and 10 I have focused on the experiences of West Indians in Britain and Canada.

A word is in order on the terminology I have used for members of various racial/geographic/residential groups—in part because the population of the West Indies is composed of different groups, and in part because there is still debate as to how people of African ancestry should define themselves. In general, I have used the term "West Indians" to refer to people of color (primarily, but not always, of African descent) from the English-speaking Caribbean who either are currently living in the West Indies or have emigrated to other countries. West Indians now residing in the United States are referred to alternately as "West Indians" or "West Indian Americans," or (when the distinction is needed) "African West Indian Americans"; persons of African descent who were born in the United States are referred to alternately as "African Americans" or "black Americans." When a distinction is needed between West Indians of African descent and the large groups in Trinidad and Guyana whose origins are in South Asia (the Indian subcontinent), I have referred to the latter as "East Indians" or "persons of East Indian descent." West Indian residents of European descent are referred to as such or as "whites"; residents of mixed African and European ancestry are referred to as "mulattos." Members of racial/geographic groups represented in the West Indies in smaller numbers are called by their specific descriptors (e.g., Chinese, Syrians, etc.).

The cases presented herein were taken both from my own clinical experience as a therapist and from the experiences of my trainees in supervision or graduate students. All names and specific details have been changed in order to maintain confidentiality.

OVERVIEW

This book is divided into three parts. Part I examines the history of the West Indies (Chapter 1), the reasons for migration (Chapter 2), West

Indian family structure (Chapter 3), educational and work values (Chapter 4), racism (Chapter 5), interisland differences (Chapter 6), and the Rastafarian culture (Chapter 7). Differences between African Americans and African West Indian Americans (Chapter 8), as well as the experience of West Indians in the United Kingdom (Chapter 9) and Canada (Chapter 10), are also addressed in this section.

Part II explores assessment (Chapter 11), issues in counseling (Chapter 12), major treatment approaches in counseling the culturally different (Chapter 13), and a model for treating West Indian families, including a case example (Chapter 14).

Part III offers training suggestions for teachers, mental health workers, speech evaluators, and parents (Chapter 15). Recommendations for future research and clinical work (Chapter 16) are also made in this section. Furthermore, the use of the West Indian Comprehensive Assessment Battery (WICAB; Appendix II) is explored in Part III. I developed the WICAB in order to assist the clinician in assessing the client's social and emotional functioning, as well as any cultural transitional conflicts the client may be experiencing as a result of migration. In addition, the WICAB compares the education systems in the West Indies and the United States, with specific references to grade equivalents, spelling differences, and skills children should have mastered given their specific grades prior to migration.

In general, *Working with West Indian Families* can be beneficial to anyone who works with West Indians. However, Parts II and III are more applicable to West Indians who have emigrated and are residing in such places as United States, Britain, and Canada, since these two sections discuss issues such as acculturation and assimilation that are not directly applicable to West Indians residing in the West Indies. But because Parts II and III focus on treatment approaches and training implications as they apply to West Indians, educators and clinicians working with families in the West Indies can also benefit from the techniques presented here.

SHARON-ANN GOPAUL-MCNICOL

Acknowledgments

Mom and Dad, throughout my life your emotional support, infinite gentleness, and unflagging confidence have been a great source of strength and an expression of your unqualified love. For always stimulating and encouraging me to reach my potential, I am deeply grateful to you.

Ulric, for the past 14 years you have supported me on my various projects, and this instance is no exception. Your intellectual curiosity has always had an infectious quality that has challenged me to seek alternative views. For giving freely of your expertise and for being an integral part of the completion of this project, I sincerely thank you.

It is true that the task of writing is often associated with neglect of those closest to us. For this reason I must thank you, Monique, for your patience and understanding. Through your own writings, I vicariously came to understand the difficulty children experience as they acclimate to this society. I feel so blessed to have had the opportunity to parent a child so warm, so loving, and so humorous. Thank you, my darling.

For the past ten years I have come to understand the true meaning of a surrogate family. I have had the support and encouragement of several people in my personal and professional life. These individuals not only read drafts of the manuscript and participated in interviews, but willingly shared their knowledge and provided comfort in trying times. The Honorable Vance Amory, Dr. Tania Thomas, and Earl George, you have brought the concept of extended family to a new level. Vance, you always took time from your busy schedule as the Premier of Nevis to resolve questions and provide constructive feedback. For your kindness and generosity, I sincerely thank you.

Tania and Earl, you have always managed to turn our scientific conversations into something more special and unique. Thank you for being my little "sister" and big "brother." A special expression of gratitude must go to my extended family: Gail, Wendy, Kurt, Nigel, Michael, Kja, Michelle, Doreen, Chris, Maria, Autricia, Vera Gibbons, and Brenda Miller. Thanks also to Drs. Lauraine Casella, Melvon Swanston, and Nicola Beckles for their support throughout this project.

While it is impossible to mention the names of all my colleagues to whom I am indebted for their critical comments and constructive suggestions, I must address special thanks to the following individuals for their important contributions to my personal and scientific development. Dr. Nancy Boyd-Franklin encouraged me to write this book. Nancy, you have been an inspiring model of scientific attitudes and clinical wisdom. Drs. Janet Brice, George Irish, Jama Adams, Delroy Louden, Carl James, Patrick Solomon, Iola Brown, Clemont London, Eleanor Armour-Thomas, Norris Haynes, Miriam Azaunce, Julia Vane, Michael Barnes, Arthur Dozier, Aldrena Mabry, and Ashton Gibson have evoked in me the epistemological and methodological rigor necessary to complete this project. I also owe a breath of thanks to Joanne Valere-Meredith, The Honorable Owen Eversley, Horace Lashley, Joannie Amory-Hypolite, Bernice Sims, Victor Jordan, Vera Weeks, Veronica Udeogalanya, Joya Gomez, Seretse McHardy, Susan Dhanoolal-Lokai, Thelma Hunkins, Geneive Brown, and Janet and Herbert Ward for their wise counsel and unintrusive support.

I thank the staff at Guilford Press, Seymour Weingarten, Editor-in-Chief, Rowena Howells, Managing Editor, and Marie Sprayberry, copy-editor, for nurturing this project and for their sound advice.

Finally I owe a profound debt to all my clients and students in training over the years. Thank you for providing me with the ideas, data, and clinical suggestions presented here. Of course, without the principals and clinicians who coordinated the groups, and the many people who willingly volunteered to be interviewed, this project may not have reached fruition. Therefore, to them I owe my deepest gratitude.

Contents

PART III. Implications

APPENDICES

PART I

HISTORICAL, EDUCATIONAL, SOCIOPOLITICAL FACTORS

CHAPTER 1

History of the
West Indies

Historically the terms "West Indies" and "the Caribbean" have been used interchangeably, since the West Indies are a group of islands stretching from the north coast of Venezuela to the south coast of Florida, situated in the Caribbean Sea.

The English-speaking Caribbean, commonly known as the British West Indies, is made up of Anguilla; Antigua and Barbuda; part of Aruba; the Bahamas; Barbados; the British Virgin Islands; the Cayman Islands; Dominica; Grenada; Jamaica; Montserrat; parts of the Netherlands Antilles; St. Christopher (St. Kitts) and Nevis; St. Lucia; St. Vincent and the Grenadines; Trinidad and Tobago; and hundreds of other smaller islands (see Appendix I). Although Belize and Guyana are not geographically in the Caribbean (Belize is in Central America and Guyana is in South America), they are part of the English-speaking Caribbean community because of their linguistic, cultural, and ethnic similarities, their economic ties, and common sociopolitical history with the British West Indies. Likewise, the U.S. Virgin Islands—St. Thomas, St. Croix, and St. John—have close links to the British West Indies because of linguistic, ethnic, and cultural commonalities.

The Spanish-speaking Caribbean islands are comprised of Cuba, the Dominican Republic, Puerto Rico, and other smaller islands. Many inhabitants of Central and South American nations (such as Panama and Costa Rica) who are of African descent and whose first home was in the Caribbean islands also have strong political, ethnic, and cultural ties to the Caribbean.

The French-speaking Caribbean encompasses Guadeloupe, Haiti, Martinique, and St. Martin. The Dutch-speaking islands are made up of parts of Aruba, St. Maarten, and parts of the Netherlands Antilles. The island of Hispaniola is shared by the Dominican Republic and Haiti. While many of the islands have gained their independence since 1962, many others are still colonies or territories of Britain (such as the British Virgin Islands), France, the Netherlands, or the United States.

For the purposes of this book, the West Indies will be defined as the English-speaking Caribbean islands plus Belize and Guyana. French-speaking Haiti will occasionally be touched on because of its tremendous contribution to the development of the Caribbean as a whole.

The West Indies is divided into the more developed countries (MDCs) and the less developed countries (LDCs). The more developed countries are Barbados, Guyana, Jamaica, and Trinidad and Tobago; the less developed countries are the remaining islands.

EARLY PEOPLE OF THE WEST INDIES

The first people in the West Indies were not of African or European heritage, but were tribes known as the Arawaks and the Caribs. These natives bore a striking resemblance to the Mongolian people of Asia, with their straight black hair, slanting eyes, and wide teeth. The Arawaks were peaceful, while the Caribs were fierce and warlike.

Before migrating to the West Indies, the Arawaks occupied the northern part of South America. As their population increased, some moved north, crossing the narrow strip of sea between what is now Venezuela and Trinidad, then going on to Cuba, Jamaica, Haiti, and the Bahamas. Meanwhile the Caribs, who were settlers of the Brazilian plateau and whose population had also increased, began to thrust outward. They first went east toward the Amazon, but later went north to Guyana and Trinidad, and along the chain of smaller islands to St. Kitts, the central part of Haiti, and Puerto Rico. There they came into contact with the peaceful Arawaks, whom they either slaughtered or drove northward. In general, the Caribs preferred the smaller islands and the Arawaks the larger ones.

EUROPEAN "DISCOVERY" OF THE WEST INDIES

Christopher Columbus, believing that the world is round and that India could be reached by sailing west, secured the backing of the

Spanish crown for an expedition to India. The purpose of this expedition (as of all others) was to secure for Spain gold, silver, pearls, and other treasures that might be found. In return, he was to be appointed viceroy, admiral, and governor-general of any new lands he "discovered." In addition, he was to receive one-eighth of the profits so derived.

On October 12, 1492, Columbus landed on one of the islands in the archipelago now known as the Bahamas. On this first voyage, he also "discovered" Cuba and Haiti. Since Columbus thought he had reached an outpost of India, he called the inhabitants "Indians." Of these natives, Columbus wrote that "all have a loving manner and a gentle speech" (Daniel, 1952, Vol. 2, p. 116). The inhabitants readily exchanged their ornaments of gold for worthless trifles such as beads, and as a result of their hospitality, Columbus made several other voyages. On his second voyage in 1493, Columbus "discovered" Jamaica, Puerto Rico, Guadeloupe, Montserrat, Antigua, St. Kitts and Nevis, St. Martin, the Virgin Islands, and several small islands. On the third voyage in 1498, he "discovered" Trinidad and Tobago, Grenada, and St. Vincent; and on his fourth voyage in 1502 he "discovered" St. Lucia, Martinique, and other small islands.

In spite of the hospitality of the natives, they were enslaved and put to work in the gold mines by Columbus and his comrades. This brutalization, along with diseases transmitted by the Europeans, proved fatal to the Arawaks, who died off rapidly and soon disappeared as a race. The Caribs, on the other hand, fiercely resisted all attempts by the Spaniards to enslave them. However, when they were carried off into slavery, they pined away and died. Despite the Caribs' strong resistance, the European weapons were superior to theirs; thus they were gradually ousted from most of the islands.

It is therefore not surprising that some West Indian artists and historians did not glorify Columbus's "discovery" of the New World during the 1992 quincentennial. Instead, the Caribbean Community (CARICOM; see below) marked 1992 as "The Encounter between Two Worlds," focusing on an examination of what the Caribbean's encounter with Europe has really meant for the past 500 years. Some organizers highlighted the genocide against the indigenous tribes, as well as the dehumanization of the African slaves and atrocities against the East Indian indentured labor. Others focused on the creative genius of the Caribbean. The major emphasis was on the fact that Columbus did not discover, but rather established contact with, the Caribbean.

THE BRITISH INFLUENCE IN THE WEST INDIES

By 1501 the entire coastline from the Amazon to the Gulf of Honduras was known to the Spaniards; throughout this area, the enslaved natives provided the labor for the mines. In 1515 Bishop Bartolome de las Casas went to Spain to plead for the natives, who were treated brutally. Finally, through his efforts, in 1542 the new "Laws of the Indies" were promulgated, abolishing Indian slavery (Daniel, 1952). However, in his attempt to spare the natives, las Casas suggested that Negroes from Africa "who were sturdy and can better endure labor on the estates and in the mines should be used for the purpose" (Daniel, 1952, Vol 2, p. 180), as they were by the Portuguese on the west coast of Africa. Thus began the notorious slave trade. It was this slave trade that brought the other Europeans, in particular the British, to the West Indies.

The African slave trade was very profitable. The main reason the English colonized the West Indies was the obvious expansive commercial and financial benefit to England. William Hawkins, "the father and founder of the slave trade" (Daniel, 1952, Vol. 2, p. 180), Francis Drake, and their successors saw no evil in this traffic. Slavery was seen as an economic necessity "for the support of the Kingdom of the Indies" (Parry, Sherlock, & Maingot, 1987, p. 17). This triangular slave trade, which continued for 400 years, began with the trip from the home port in England to Africa, and then continued to the West Indies. It was only through slavery that the British were able to cultivate their estates. Thus "the West Indian islands became the hub of the British Empire, of immense importance to the grandeur and prosperity of England" (Williams, 1967).

Other European nations, including the French (from 1528) and the Dutch (from 1632), later participated in the African slave trade. They also established colonies in the West Indies, dividing these lands among themselves. Some islands in the West Indies are still colonies and are still referred to as the British, French, or Dutch West Indies.

THE ABOLITION OF SLAVERY AND THE POSTEMANCIPATION PERIOD

In 1833 a bill was introduced in the British Parliament to abolish slavery in the British West Indies. However, this was only to take effect from 1840; during the intervening years a system of apprenticeship, intended to help the slaves gradually adjust to the new order of things, was to be implemented. But the apprenticeship period proved little better than slavery, since the planters were determined to wring the last ounce of labor out of the apprentices before complete emancipation. It is important to remember that the West Indian islands had come to be extremely important to the British economy.

Although slavery had ended, the government remained in the hands of the old landowners, and the colonizers still continued class oppression. The educational, social, and political systems in the West Indies were all fashioned after the British system. The carving up of the West Indian region by the Spanish, British, French, and Dutch and the conscious supplanting of the African culture was the beginning of a lack of identity and a constant fascination by the West Indian people with what is European and white.

THE UNITED STATES IN THE CARIBBEAN

In 1823 President James Monroe espoused the Monroe Doctrine, which, in essence, stated that the United States opposed further European colonization or intervention in the Western Hemisphere. Influenced by this Monroe Doctrine, the United States unilaterally exercised economic and military power in the Caribbean. During the second half of the nineteenth century, the Caribbean became the main site of American expansion. By the beginning of the twentieth century, the United States had become the most powerful industrial country in the world, partly because of its economic penetration of the Caribbean.

In 1903 President Theodore Roosevelt, recognizing the strategic value of a canal across the isthmus of Panama, exploited the discontent between the Panamanians and Colombians (at this time Panama was a part of Colombia), eventually proclaiming Panama an independent republic and the United States as its protectorate. Since the government of Panama was new and uncertain of itself, there was no protest against this arrangement, nor against the Canal Treaty that was hastily drafted by the American government. By this treaty, the United States government was granted in perpetuity a strip of Panamanian territory over which it could exercise complete control. President Roosevelt attempted to justify this arrangement by the nineteenth-century doctrine of "manifest destiny"—that is, the belief that the United States expansion to the Pacific coast was inevitable, since the world benefited from these measures.

The history of U.S. involvement in the Caribbean can be divided into four phases. In the early twentieth century, American policy can be thought of as the "big stick" policy because of aggression toward the developing Caribbean nations. From about 1912 to early 1930, the U.S. policy in the Caribbean can be seen as "dollar diplomacy." During this era, the United States pumped dollars into countries that were politically and economically unstable, in the hope of bringing about stability. But by this time, the American image was stained in the Caribbean. In an attempt to remedy this tarnished image, the United States inaugurated the "good neighbor" policy. Thus acts of aggression were reduced and U.S. rights to intervention were surrendered. However, with the advent of the Cold War in 1945, followed by the success of the Cuban revolution and the emergence of communist and socialist political leaders, the "good neighbor" policy was discarded. From the 1950s to the 1990s, the United States shifted its energy to discouraging the spread of communism and socialism in the Caribbean.

U.S. involvement in the English-speaking Caribbean came in the aftermath of World War II. As British control declined, and as several Caribbean islands became independent from 1960 onward, the United States became the main source of economic assistance to the region. In February 1982, in his address to the Organization of American States, President Reagan stated that the Caribbean "is a vital strategic and commercial artery for the United States. Nearly half of U.S. trade, two-thirds of our imported oil, and over half of imported strategic minerals pass through the region" (Stewart, 1986, p. 1). In providing economic assistance to the Caribbean, the United States used the strategies of punishment and reward. Countries that pursued policies inimical to the interests of the United States did not receive economic aid (e.g., Guyana and Jamaica from 1974 to 1978 and Grenada from 1980 to 1983); countries whose policies were congruent with those of the United States did receive aid (e.g., Jamaica from 1981 to the present). Thus U.S. policy in the Caribbean derives from both factors related to critical U.S. interests—economic and political security.

THE WEST INDIAN FEDERATION AND CARICOM

The British emerged from World War II so exhausted and financially drained that they were unable to continue their imperial adventures. Britain had to contend with a massive domestic reconstruction that did not allow it to channel resources into West Indian dependencies. In addition, the British government did not want to be responsible for either unproductive sugar plantations or a large, uneducated underclass. Thus independence was thrust upon the West Indian people because Britain was no longer able to act as a "mother country" to these islands. Many feared that independence would mean a decline in their standard of living because of the withdrawal of British funds.

Faced with the prospect of independence, several islands formed a West Indian Federation on January 3, 1958, with the hope that they would unite and maximize their economic and political power. Unfortunately, the federation came into existence in the face of very strong island loyalties and jealousies, which reflected a considerable diversity in social and economic origins as well as in political development. People of the different islands had little knowledge of each other because of the cultural fragmentation created by the dividing up of the islands among their former "mother countries." Jamaica and Trinidad and Tobago (the more economically developed of the islands) felt they would be responsible for carrying the burden of the less developed countries. In addition, none of these colonies had ever been taught the principles of self-government. Thus these weakly structured countries were unable at that time to form a linkage with respect to educational, social, and political administration. Each country was focusing on its own internal development. Jamaica was the first to pull out; the then premier of Trinidad and Tobago said, "One from ten leaves nought," so Trinidad and Tobago pulled out. The West Indian Federation collapsed in 1962, after four years of seeking to work out an accommodation among the ten Caribbean governments that had been parties to the experiment. Most of the effort during the four years had been devoted, understandably, to political questions. When the federation collapsed, it left behind feelings of resentment because, as Eric Williams (1981) stated, "any federation is better than no federation" (p. 285). However, the value in regional cooperation, especially from an economic and commercial standpoint, had also been noted. (Jamaica achieved independence on August 6, 1962; Trinidad and Tobago on August 31, 1962; and St. Kitts and Nevis on September 19, 1983.) In a sense, the end of the federation came to be regarded as the real beginning of what is now the CARICOM. In July 1965, the Caribbean Free Trade Association (CARIFTA) was formed. In July 1973, CARIFTA was transformed into a Common Market that became an integral part of CARICOM. Currently the members of CARICOM are Antigua and Barbuda, the Bahamas, Barbados, Belize, Dominica, Grenada, Guyana, Jamaica, Montserrat, St. Kitts and Nevis, St. Lucia, St. Vincent and the Grenadines, and Trinidad and Tobago, with other islands having observer status. The objectives are to attain economic cooperation through the Caribbean Common Market and to have common services in functional matters such as health, education, culture, communications, and industrial relations.

THE NEED FOR A REGIONAL WEST INDIAN IDENTITY

A major problem facing the West Indies today is a lack of a true West Indian identity and the continued involvement of external influences (Ambursley & Cohen, 1983). This may be the result of two factors—continued psychological colonialism and a narrow-minded nationalism. Each country is seeking a new national identity, a new national flag, a new national anthem, new national heroes and heroines. For territories so small and lacking in resources, however, a narrow-minded political nationalism can result in political suicide. Political regional anarchy and economic self-destruction are rife in the West Indies today. Each island is trying to win the favor of the United States at the expense of regional unification. To attain a true West Indian perspective, economic stability, and a broader political nationalism, they must all surrender this provincial insularity for a new regional identity and cooperate in areas of mutual need. As Eugenia Charles (1991), Dominica's Prime Minister, stated,

> . . . let us not delude ourselves that our interests lie in the big league. Most of us are but fledglings in the game of international politics and trade. Until we begin to see the Caribbean as one region, one market, we will forever be pulling at straws. (p. 26)

CURRENT DEMOGRAPHICS OF WEST INDIANS IN THE WEST INDIES

West Indians are a heterogeneous group of people whose customs have been influenced by African, Spanish, British, French, Dutch, Asian, and American cultures. With the exception of Trinidad and Guyana, people of African heritage make up about 90% of the population in most of the islands. European and American whites make up about 5%, and Chinese and mulattos (persons of mixed African and European descent) make up the remaining 5%.

In Trinidad and Guyana, East Indians make up about 41% of the population, with those of African descent also constituting about 41% and whites, Chinese, and mulattos the remaining 18%. The native inhabitants who managed to survive later intermingled with the African slaves, so that today the indigenous people of the West Indies are practically nonexistent.

The people of the West Indies are predominantly Christians, with the East Indians in Trinidad and Guyana being primarily Hindus or Muslims.

CHAPTER 2

Migration

In 1985, the New York City Department of Planning, Office of Immigrant Affairs and Population Analysis Division, released a paper entitled "Caribbean Immigrants in New York City: A Demographic Summary." Based mainly on 1980 U.S. census data, the paper indicated that Caribbean immigrants accounted for 28% (470,000) of the foreign-born residing in New York City. This figure includes people from all islands of the British, French, and Dutch West Indies, as well as the ethnically and culturally related countries of Guyana and Panama; it excludes people from the American Caribbean islands, such as Puerto Rico and the U.S. Virgin Islands. The Immigration and Naturalization Service (INS) adjustment data for the 1990 census suggested that this number would have doubled by 1990. According to the New York City Department of Planning, exact figures for 1990 will not be available until 1993.

Data for INS fiscal years 1983 through 1987 showed that 40.4% (173,693) of the immigrants in New York City granted permanent resident alien status were from the Caribbean: 22.3% were English, French, or Dutch speakers from the West Indies, and 18.1% were Spanish speakers from Cuba or the Dominican Republic. It must be borne in mind that these figures include only those who responded to the census. The actual numbers were probably much larger, since most undocumented aliens were not counted. The Department of Planning believes, on the basis of school enrollment, that the ratio of documented to undocumented Caribbeans in New York State alone is 1:1.

The influx of Caribbean citizens to the United States began about 1900, when a severe depression in the Caribbean sugar industry was triggered by the introduction of European beet sugar. With the World

War II labor shortage, many workers migrated to the United States from the British West Indies, with the largest percentage coming from Jamaica (because of its geographic proximity), followed by Trinidad, Barbados, and Grenada. Most Caribbean immigrants settled in New York State, with more than half settling in New York City. Caribbean immigration continued in the postwar decades, major contributing factors being geographic proximity, poverty and unemployment in the home countries, and the fact that in 1962 Britain closed its doors to immigration from the black Commonwealth countries.

Resident alien status is usually granted to immediate relatives (spouses, children, parents) of U.S. citizens, refugees, and special immigrants. Individuals with resident alien status are better able to integrate into the social fabric of the society than are illegal immigrants. While the employment sector is open only to legal residents, thrusting undocumented (illegal) residents into menial, off-the-books jobs, the school system and the public health sector are open to both legal and illegal residents. Some immigrants are unaware of this; others do not enroll their children in school or seek health services out of fear of being deported.

GENDER, AGE, AND MARITAL STATUS OF IMMIGRANTS

Traditionally, migration from the West Indies was dominated by young males (Marshall, 1982). Since 1960 migration has been dominated by females because of the types of jobs available at the destinations—for example, jobs as domestics, nurse's aides, and health aides, all female-dominated growth industries. These women establish networks that serve as a support for newly arrived immigrants, with families and friends settling in the same communities.

Today, Caribbean immigrants generally tend to cluster in the 15–29 age bracket, with immigrants from the British, French, or Dutch West Indies mainly in the 25–29 age group (New York City Department of Planning, 1985).

Approximately 50.5% of West Indian immigrants to the United States are married, with men slightly more likely than women to be so (New York City Department of Planning, 1985).

SOCIOECONOMIC CLASS OF WEST INDIAN IMMIGRANTS

Most immigrants are from the lower or middle socioeconomic classes; they come to the United States "for a better life" or to "educate our children." Because of the limited national resources in most West Indian countries, high schools can accommodate only a minority of students. Thus children have to take an entrance examination in order to go to a government high school. In Jamaica, only 25% of potential students obtain a free high school education. For the other islands the percentages range from 30% to 40%, except for the very small islands, where the population is so small that all students receive a free high school education. The problem, of course, is what happens to the remaining 60% to 75% of the students. In fact, "the majority receive some other type of secondary education and the phenomenon is associated with the socioeconomic background of parents" (Clarke & Bolarinde, 1989, p. 3). These new secondary schools, which accommodate those who were "unsuccessful" on the entrance examination, "offer programs which are 20% academic and 80% vocational" (Clarke & Bolarinde, 1989, p. 3). The focus is on skill training, both for these students and for the adolescents who do not attend any school and receive, at most, worksite training. Thus, for students with academic/career aspirations, there is no place in West Indian societies unless their parents are affluent enough to afford private schools. But even people who might have held relatively good government jobs (teachers, counselors, etc.) in their homelands may migrate because it is so difficult to accumulate wealth, given the low salaries and high cost of living.

Usually when people from the upper echelons of the society migrate, they do so to acquire advanced education. In many instances, they return to their native lands on completion of their schooling abroad.

INTENDED RESIDENCE AND OCCUPATION

From 1983 through 1987 New York City received 95,783 documented West Indian immigrants. The majority of West Indian immigrants live in Brooklyn (58.8%), followed by Queens (18.1%), the Bronx (17.2%), Manhattan (5.6%), and Staten Island (0.4%). In New York City, there is a tendency for them to live in enclaves, the largest pockets being in Brooklyn's Crown Heights and Flatbush (New York City Department of Planning, 1985), whereas in Los Angeles "few live in proximity to fellow countrymen" (Justus, 1983, p. 4).

Most West Indian immigrants in New York City who are employed work in the service sector, followed by employment areas designated "precision, craft, and repair" and "operator, fabricator, and laborer," followed by "administrative support" and "professional and technical" (New York City Department of Planning, 1985).

IMMIGRATION LAWS

Immigrants arrive in the United States under a system of preferences involving family ties, job skills, and other criteria. Some categories most applicable to West Indians are the following (P.L. 101-649 Immigration Act of 1990):

1. Permanent residents—those who hold green cards—are legal residents who are permitted to work, receive Social Security, and receive unemployment benefits. The only limitation is that permanent residents are unable to vote or to hold federal jobs.

2. Conditional permanent residents are primarily spouses of legal residents.

3. Nonimmigrants are temporary workers, students, visitors, and so forth. They are expected to return to their home countries upon expiration of their visas.

4. Undocumented or illegal aliens are in the United States without a satisfactory immigration status, either temporary or permanent. An estimated 3 to 4 million people are in the country illegally. Many West Indians fall into this category and are thus unable to hold legal jobs. They tend to live privately, drawing little attention to themselves, for fear of being deported. This fear makes them vulnerable to extortion and other abuse, including sexual abuse of women.

5. Refugees are persons fleeing persecution because of their race, religion, ethnicity, political opinion, or membership in a particular social group. Haitians and Cubans have traditionally received refugee status more often than any other Caribbean groups.

6. Political asylees are refugees who are present in the United States at the time they apply for refugee protection. Those granted asylum are entitled to certain refugee benefits.

7. Legalized aliens were granted amnesty under the Immigration Reform and Control Act of 1986 either by virtue of continuous illegal residence in the United States prior to January 1, 1982, or by having performed agricultural work.

Employment-based immigration provides entry for "priority workers" (aliens with extraordinary ability in the sciences, the arts, business, athletics, etc.); workers capable of performing skilled labor for which qualified U.S. workers are not available; certain special immigrants (such as ministers); and individuals with a certain amount of money to invest in an enterprise that will create at least ten jobs for U.S. workers.

On November 29, 1990, President Bush signed into law the Immigration Act of 1990 (P.L. 101-649), which in many ways creates the most comprehensive system of immigration regulations in the nation's history and effects significant changes since the 1965 Immigration Act. The numerous changes made by this law went into effect October 1, 1991. Many undocumented immigrants are not aware of their rights and are therefore taken advantage of by others. Although undocumented immigrants have few rights compared to permanent residents and U.S. citizens, it is important for undocumented immigrants to know and exercise those that do exist. The legal rights of undocumented immigrants include the following (P.L. 101-649):

1. Immigrants have the right to refuse to allow an immigration agent into their homes, answer any questions, or show the agent any documents if the agent does not have a valid search warrant. If the agent enters a home by force or without a search warrant, the immigrant should contact an attorney immediately.

2. An immigrant who is stopped or detained on the street by an immigration agent has the right to remain silent, which an undocumented alien should do. An immigrant who is arrested should give the agent no information, since it can be used against the immigrant in deportation proceedings, but should insist on speaking to an attorney. After an arrest, the INS must provide a list of attorneys who will provide free legal services if the immigrant cannot afford to pay a private attorney.

3. In order to enter an immigrant's place of work, an immigration agent must have a valid search or arrest warrant or the employer's permission. If the agent enters by force to make an arrest, the immigrant should remain silent and demand to speak to an attorney.

4. Immigrants should not sign their names on any document without speaking to an attorney. By signing a document, they may be giving up certain rights (waiver) or agreeing to return to their home countries (voluntary departure).

5. Public schools are obliged to admit all children, regardless of their immigration status. Public schools should not ask for children's or parents' immigration status.

6. Publicly funded hospitals are required to provide emergency medical services, regardless of the patient's immigration status. Immigration status generally does not affect a pregnant woman's

eligibility for Medicaid. Undocumented parents can apply for public benefits and Medicaid for a child who is a citizen of the United States.

7. All workers, including the undocumented, are entitled by law to join or organize a labor union. Employers are forbidden by law to break a union-organizing effort by calling in the INS.

8. Undocumented workers are eligible to receive unemployment insurance, workers' compensation, and disability benefits when they and the employer have contributed to the fund. However, an undocumented worker is not eligible for Social Security retirement benefits (even if the employer deducts money from the worker's pay to contribute to the Social Security program), unless he or she has work authorization. Immigrants who wish to know more about their rights should contact the Center for Immigrant Rights, whose address and telephone number are given in Appendix VI.

PSYCHOSOCIAL FACTORS IN MIGRATION THAT AFFECT ACCULTURATION

This section focuses on the general process of migration and acculturation as it pertains to West Indian immigrants. Berry, Minde, Kim, and Mok (1987) define acculturation as a "culture change which results from continuous first hand contact between two distinct cultural groups" (p. 494). This really involves a "shift in the cultural emphasis," involving "people in a relationship to an environment that is changing or changed" (Fabrega, 1969, p. 316). Acculturation can be examined from many perspectives, including the educational, economic, class, cultural, psychological, behavioral, and so forth. Thus an educated individual who voluntarily decided to migrate and intends to assimilate and adopt the values of the host country may experience less acculturational stress. All immigrants, however, face a period of adjustment, for immigration itself is "a process that stimulates mixed and varied responses at unpredictable periods of time" (Arredondo-Down, 1981, p. 376). Immigrants can experience a sense of loss, sadness, and disorientation, as well as feelings of happiness and exhilaration.

Berry and associates (1987) propose five stages of acculturation:

1. *Physical changes.* The individual must cope with living in a new place, including such elements as increased population density and more pollution.
2. *Biological changes.* The individual encounters, for example, a new nutritional status and new diseases.

3. *Cultural changes.* Political, economic, technical, linguistic, religious, and social institutions become altered, or new ones take their place.
4. *New sets of social relationships.* The individual must function within new social networks, both ingroup and outgroup.
5. *Psychological and behavioral changes.* An alteration in mental health status resulting from culture shock almost always occurs in some form or the other as individuals attempt to adapt to their new milieu.

Oberg (1972, cited in Arredondo-Down, 1981) proposes five stages in the process of culture shock with respect to immigrants:

1. The immigrants feel euphoria about the exciting new culture.
2. Failure to succeed leads to extreme dissatisfaction with the host culture. This is a period of psychological transition from back-home values to host-home values.
3. Persons begin to understand the host culture and feel more in touch with themselves.
4. The host culture is viewed as offering both positive and negative alternatives.
5. The immigrants return home and experience reverse culture shock.

Like most immigrants, West Indians experience acculturational stress and culture shock. Some factors that may either mitigate or exacerbate the stress and shock are prior intercultural experiences, voluntariness of migration, education, racism, and social support systems.

Prior intercultural experiences, such as having lived in an urban setting, play an important role. West Indians who migrated first to the United Kingdom and then to the United States tend to assimilate better because of the prior experience of living elsewhere.

People who were forced to leave their native countries (a "push" factor) in order to escape from unpleasant situations, such as poverty, political repression, or personal problems, tend to have greater difficulty in adjusting. Those who left to study abroad or to achieve greater personal growth (a "pull" factor) tend to experience less acculturational stress.

Education appears to be a consistent predictor of low stress (Berry et al., 1987). One reason may be that education is usually European-oriented, thus offering some acculturation prior to the actual contact with the new country. In addition, more education may allow an individual to view the change in culture as a challenge rather than a stressor. Chapter 5 discusses the effect of racism on acculturation.

Social support factors have also been found to correlate with low stress in acculturation. Legal immigrants have more access to social support networks than illegal immigrants, who have to establish their own support networks. Churches serve as good support systems in the areas of interpersonal, emotional, and religious needs. Moreover, people who have been able to establish contact with and participate in the larger society tend to have less stress in acculturation.

Like most immigrants initially, West Indian immigrants "have two lives, one back home and one here. It adds up to almost no life" (Rimer, 1991, p. B6-L). The goal when they come here is to "save money, buy a house back home and go back and start a business" (Rimer, 1991, p. B6-L). However, going back is harder than they anticipated because it is quite difficult for them to attain their goals; they live here physically, but remain emotionally in their homelands. Many of them have the responsibility to repay family members back home who assisted in their migration. Some migrants, especially undocumented ones, must work two jobs to meet their responsibilities both back home and in the new country. The children have enormous problems because their parents have little time to assist in their adjustment. They are expected simultaneously to assimilate and to maintain and respect their parents' traditional cultural values; they too are expected to live between two worlds. In addition, initially the families live in crowded conditions (normally with relatives or friends), making it difficult for children to concentrate on their studies.

Although it is necessary to assist immigrant families in their adjustment by mitigating acculturational stress, because "too much stress may inhibit effective response to acculturation" (Berry et al., 1987, p. 508), it is important to remember the Yerkes–Dodson law, which states that some level of acculturational stress is needed to alert a person to impending dangers. Thus a curvilinear relationship between arousal and performance is necessary to attain optimal level of acculturation.

In assessing the degree of acculturation, the West Indian Comprehensive Assessment Battery (WICAB; see Appendix II) can be used at an early stage in therapy. Although no score is obtained from this assessment tool, it is a comprehensive measure for ascertaining how a West Indian immigrant is assimilating into this society. Simply bringing into consciousness (for both the therapist and the client) the problems that the family members are experiencing, and examining solutions and possible options, are ways of providing some direction.

Establishing goals and objectives in therapy will be facilitated by using such a comprehensive assessment measure.

In general, the WICAB addresses parent–child relationships—for instance, children's relationships with parents whom they might not have seen for several years during a separation period before the children migrated. Racial attitude, self-concept, social relations, academic goals, psychological functioning, work/school adjustment, support systems, acculturative stress, and overall cultural adjustment are all explored via the WICAB. In addition, specific measures such as the Immigrant Self-Concept Scale (see Appendix III) can be a useful measure in determining in exactly what area an immigrant's self-concept is poor. Chapters 11 and 12 can be of further assistance in assessing West Indian families and providing therapeutic intervention.

CHAPTER 3

The West Indian Family

This chapter describes the typical family organization and structure in the West Indies. The data were collected by means of the Immigrant Self-Concept Scale (Appendix III), the West Indian Attitude Survey (Appendix V), and the Immigrant Attitude Survey (Appendix IV), which were randomly distributed to 792 people of West Indian backgrounds in the United States, the United Kingdom, and Canada, as well as to native residents of several islands in the West Indies (notably, Jamaica, Trinidad and Tobago, Barbados, Grenada, St. Vincent and the Grenadines, St. Kitts and Nevis, and St. Lucia). Although the family organization described in this chapter may not exactly reflect family roles and dynamics in Jamaica, most of the other islands of the West Indies share a family structure like the one described here. For a more detailed examination of interisland differences, see Chapter 6.

FAMILY ROLES

Cohen (1956) identifies four types of family organization in the West Indies: (1) "The Christian family" is based on formal marriage and a patriarchal order approximating that of Christian families in other parts of the world. This family structure, which carries much status, is more frequently seen among the middle and upper classes. (2) "The faithful concubinage" (called "living" in Trinidad), also based on a patriarchal order, has no legal status but is a well-established union of at least three years' duration. Although these unions are not regularized by a civil or religious ceremony, they tend to be culturally and officially accepted. The couple may have children, and they tend to be seen in the community as a family. The man lives with the woman as if he were married to her and performs all the functions of a legal spouse. (3) "The companionate family" describes individuals who are living together primarily for pleasure and convenience, usually for a period of less than three years. (4) "The disintegrated family" consists of women and children only, in which men merely visit the women from time to time. The advantage of the last three family structures is that the woman does not feel that she is unduly dominated by her man.

Within the nuclear family structure, "the man's primary responsibilities are economic. As the head of the household, he is expected to support his wife and their children. A husband failing to provide for his family is seen as not fulfilling his role and this is grounds for divorce" (Brice, 1982, p. 128).

Although there has been an increase in the number of working women since the 1980s, a West Indian woman's primary responsibility is still childrearing. It is she who takes care of the home, and as the mother, she is clearly the nurturant figure. As a result, matters involving the children reflect upon her self-esteem. However, her role is not limited to the children; traditionally, she is also the caretaker of her husband, preparing his meals, mending his clothes, basically taking care of all his needs. In other words, a man expects of his wife very much what he expected of his mother.

The result of this arrangement is that women assume power behind the scenes while outwardly supporting their husbands' authority. This arrangement can work as long as a wife does not challenge her husband and as long as she is not expected to assume his role. Here lies the problem in migration, since the roles of men and women are often reversed. When a family migrates because of economic need, the woman may assume the role of breadwinner, thereby encroaching on her husband's main role. Unless both parties can accept this change and respect their new roles, conflicts will occur. Often the wife becomes resentful because she is still expected to perform all the domestic duties in spite of having a full-time job. The demand on the husband to share his breadwinner role may result in family dysfunction. The man may feel that his authority is being undermined by his wife's new role, and may sense a lack of respect from his wife and children because he is unable to fulfill the traditional responsibilities of a husband and a father. Feeling inadequate and emasculated, especially if his wife openly challenges his authority, the man may distance himself from any family involvement and displace his frustration and anger onto his family. If the husband is unable to regain his dominant position through employment, he may experience panic and confusion. The wife in turn may develop contempt for her husband because he is no longer fulfilling his "manly duties." Marital separation is quite common in such instances. Chapters 11 and 12 discuss this issue in more detail.

THE EXTENDED FAMILY

The West Indian family is usually an extended family that encompasses not only those related by marriage and blood, but also godparents, adopted children whose adoption is informal ("child lending"), and in some cases even friends. The function of these nonrelated family members is to provide security for children and to offer help in crises. It is common practice to give a child as a companion to an aunt, a sister, a childless woman, or a woman whose children have left home. The extended family is a source of strength for the couple; without this additional support, stress and tension may result. It is particularly useful for women, who may rely on other women in the extended family for help with childrearing and household duties. Without such support, a wife may feel her tasks are insurmountable and expect her husband to assist her, which in turn may lead to resentment on his part; arguments, drinking, gambling, and affairs may be the consequences. The extended family also serves as a measure of control against violence, with family members intervening in spouses' arguments and offering advice to them.

MARRIAGE

Marriage is marked not only by the creation of a new family but also by the continuation of the man's family line. The woman changes her name to his, even if she is a professional woman (although it is common today for women to use hyphenated names). Because traditionally a person does not marry without the blessing of the family, sons in general marry women of whom their parents, especially their mothers, approve.

Some causes of marital tension are lack of communication and sexual problems. Modern Western societies value open expression of ideas and feelings. Everyone is encouraged to speak his or her mind, even children and women, since openness and honesty are desirable attributes. However, in West Indian society, there is a different attitude toward open communication of thoughts and feelings. Several factors influence the manner in which individuals communicate. Gender, age, social and marital status, parenthood (i.e., whether one has a child), educational level, and occupation all determine who will initiate conversation, speak more vociferously, maintain eye contact or look away, change the subject, and so forth—in summary, who will dominate and who will accommodate. Thus men usually communicate directly, whereas women often talk around the point. Women tend to avoid directness and confrontation, and often do not tell their spouses exactly what is bothering them. Miscommunication, frustration, and anger result, because the women do not feel that their husbands understand or are sensitive to their needs.

Feelings such as love are frequently not openly expressed. Love is usually expressed only to infants, at times to the point of indulgence. Thus in the Eriksonian (Erikson, 1980) sense, the child develops a sense of basic trust. But as the infant becomes a young child, affection is no longer as openly exhibited. Instead, love is traditionally affirmed through certain actions, such as the father's hard work to provide for the family and the mother's caring for a child's basic needs.

West Indian women are taught to sublimate or repress their sexual drives and tend to consider sex as an obligation. From birth, girls are taught to be modest, which causes embarrassment about their bodies. So when a woman marries, she is expected to be ignorant about sex and is expected to be more concerned about being a good mother than a good sexual partner to her husband (Henry & Wilson, 1975). In fact, women, especially those of the middle and upper classes, are expected to be virgins when entering consensual unions. On the other hand, men are expected to know all about sex before they marry. This double standard continues after marriage: Men more freely engage in extramarital affairs, while women are expected to be faithful.

Traditionally women marry between the ages of 22 and 27, while men marry in their late 20s or early 30s. Divorce is not common; couples may separate for many years and never divorce. Likewise abortion is not commonly viewed as a viable option for an unwanted pregnancy; it is, in fact, illegal, although some doctors will perform abortions privately. Even if couples separate, men are expected to support their children. While some of them do so, most are unable to because they are unemployed. In such cases, the woman's family assists her financially in caring for her children.

ROLES OF CHILDREN

Respect is a core value in West Indian society. For children to be disrespectful to their parents assaults the very heart of the parent–child relationship. Respect for authority is learned in the home and reinforced in the community and in the school. The hierarchy is clearly defined. Although parents and children may love and respect one another, parents generally do not aspire to be friends with their children. A child who calls an adult by his or her first name is seen as disrespectful. Children must use titles, such as "Mr." or "Mrs.," "Aunt" or "Uncle." It is considered impolite for a child to contradict an elder. Younger siblings are expected to respect and obey their older brothers and sisters in the absence of their parents; conversely, older children are expected to help their parents care for their younger siblings or their grandparents.

During late childhood and throughout adolescence, children are expected to perform household chores with no expectation of rewards. Feelings of obligation govern much of the traditional life of families. Shame and open reprimand among family members are frequently used to reinforce adherence to familial obligations. Little emphasis is put on self-reliance, as in the U.S. society. In contrast, it is felt that people are only what they are through the efforts of many other individuals. Thus obligation is a crucial concept, be it spoken or unspoken. Everyone understands the hierarchical nature of relationships: A child has an obligation to his or her parents, teachers, and employer, with the greatest obligation being to one's parents. This debt is owed forever and is never truly repaid. Regardless of what parents do, children are obliged to respect and obey them. Needless to say, when such a child comes into contact with U.S. society—with its emphasis on self-sufficiency, being the master of one's own destiny, and doing one's own thing—he or she can at times experience much conflict, stress, and anxiety.

To this day, there are differences in the way males and females in the West Indies are socialized. The most important child is the oldest son. Like the father, he commands more respect and receives better treatment. He is expected to be a role model for his siblings not only in childhood but throughout life. When the father dies, he becomes the leader in the family. If he abdicates this role, either by outrightly refusing it or by behaving irresponsibly, the next son fills it. Boys are encouraged to be achievers, to pursue academics, and to seek respectable professions.

Girls are taught all domestic responsibilities so that they can be good wives and mothers. They are expected to be pretty, obedient, unassertive, sexually nonalluring, and respectful of themselves. In spite of the first son's being an important figure among his siblings, it is the eldest daughter who is, to a large extent, the "parental" child. It is she who shoulders more domestic responsibilities in the absence of the parents.

Parents tend to have a relaxed attitude toward certain developmental milestones. A child who does not walk or talk by a particular age is not pressured to do so or viewed with concern. Parents can talk comfortably, for example, about a child being slow or not yet toilet-trained. Thus there is a great acceptance of a child's individuality.

In general, mother–child relations are strong, particularly the mother–son relationship. In fact, the closeness in the mother–son relationship continues even after the son is married. The son's wife is expected to understand that her husband has to care for his mother in addition to his new family. Traditionally, there has been little expectation that women will care for adult parents; this attitude is changing somewhat, as more women are employed in the workforce.

If not as close to their children as mothers are, West Indian fathers still manage to maintain affectionate and warm relations with their offspring. The major potential setback to this closeness can be the family's economic situation. Economically deprived families require that the fathers seek employment anywhere that jobs are available. This may mean a long daily commute or living elsewhere during the week and coming home only on weekends. This is more commonly the case in the larger countries such as Guyana, Jamaica, and Trinidad and Tobago.

In general, children are not encouraged to seek employment outside the home. However, as they become young adults, they must contribute one-third to one-half of their earnings to the home for their room and board. Adult children tend to stay at home until they get married. This is not perceived as immature and irresponsible, as it often is in the United States. In contrast, leaving home to live on one's own before marriage is perceived as a more deviant act than staying at home. Whereas unmarried adult males can come and go as they please, unmarried adult females are still accountable to parental rules and regulations. Mothers tend to feel embarrassed when their daughters reach age 30 and are still unmarried. The young woman is referred to as an "old maid" and is seen as "barren" because she is childless. No such stigma is placed on the unmarried adult male, who is seen as taking his time to choose a wife or is called a "sweet man," especially if he has many ladies.

LIVING ARRANGEMENTS

In general, adult males and females sleep in the same room. This is primarily because of an economic situation that forces several people from an extended family to reside in the same house. It is not unusual for boys and girls to sleep in the same bed as young children. Needless to say, families experience cultural shock when they come to the United States and are told this act can be construed as incestuous. This is not to say that incest does not occur; father–daughter incest is the deviant sexual act most often practiced, followed by uncle–niece and brother–sister incest. Because of the strong concept of family secrecy—the sentiment that "our business must stay in the home"—incest, spousal abuse, and other family problems are kept within the family. It is only within the last few years that Caribbeans have begun to examine these serious matters from social, psychological, educational, and legal perspectives.

DISCIPLINE

During the first three or four years of a child's life, the father is not generally a direct source of either emotional gratification or punishment (as male and female roles change, this tradition is slowly waning). After this age, the father begins to administer punishment, but only at the instigation of the mother. In general, parents often speak harshly to their children. They ask a question and then answer it themselves, complaining that a child refused to answer even though he or she did not have a chance to speak. Corporal punishment, such as spanking, is an acceptable form of discipline. Children are slapped or beaten with a switch merely for being disobedient, for breaking something (even accidentally) or for dawdling while on an errand. Since corporal punishment is an acceptable form of discipline, these actions are not perceived as child abuse by the family. Many West Indian families are amazed when they are charged with child abuse by the legal system. I recall one father who was prepared to go to court and attempt to convince the judge that children are better off being spanked. The adage "To spare the rod is to spoil the child" is endorsed by many.

Although the mother is the main disciplinarian, the father is in fact the real enforcer. The mother is expected to support the father's disciplinary measures. However, although she does this in his presence, covertly she may disagree with him at times and, in his absence, may be more permissive of certain behaviors of which he does not approve. Thus the children request of her things they may not ask of their father. At such times the mother's role is that of a mediator between the children and their father, and the father may soften his position as a result of the mother's mediation rather than the child's persuasion. In West Indian society, it is important to recognize that the mother's centrality is usually reinforced. At times the mother forms such a strong alliance with the children that the father feels isolated, which results in anger and conflict in the home.

CHAPTER 4

Education and Work Values

THE PLACING OF WEST INDIAN CHILDREN IN SCHOOL

Educating West Indian children poses a challenge to U.S. public schools, which must take into consideration West Indian culture as part of their multicultural curricula. The major problem facing educators, however, is the placement of these children in their correct grades upon entry into the school system. McNicol (1991) has cautioned parents about the possibility of their children's being demoted upon entering the U.S. school system. This, of course, may result in a child's losing interest in school because of boredom.

Part 2 of the WICAB (Appendix II) compares the terminology used to designate grades in different West Indian countries to that of the United States. In some countries, such as Jamaica, the same grade numbers are used at the elementary level as in the United States. In other countries, such as Trinidad and Tobago, different numerals and terminologies are used. So whereas in Jamaica and the United States a 10-year-old child is in Grade 5, in Trinidad the child is in Standard 4. There is no system of junior high school in the West Indies. While 12-year-olds in some parts of the United States (those not employing a "middle school" system) enter junior high school, those in the West Indies enter high school. Thus West Indian students can spend seven years in the same high school before going on to university. The last year of high school in the West Indies is equivalent to the first year of college in the United States. In the West Indies the term "university" is used to describe the academic institution beyond high school; in the United States the term "college" is used. Many West Indian parents experience confusion when they are told their children will be going to college as opposed to university, because some high schools in the West Indies are called colleges. Once differences in terminology are understood, placing a child in his or her correct grade should be quite simple.

Of course, it is always best to administer an educational screening test to determine West Indian children's skills relative to those their U.S. peers. This should aid educators in developing a remediation plan if needed, particularly in the areas of mathematics and reading. McNicol (1991) discusses the difficulty West Indian children face when they realize that some words are spelled differently in the United States than in the West Indies, a topic discussed in some detail in Chapter 11. It is recommended that a transcript from the child's previous school be requested, since this aids in the transition. Elsewhere, my colleagues and I (Gopaul-McNicol, Thomas, & Irish, 1991) provide a simple checklist for parents of what to bring with them when migrating to the United States; we also discuss educational and social issues that immigrants should know about in order to make a smooth adjustment to the U.S. system.

THE VALUE OF EDUCATION IN THE WEST INDIES

For the typical West Indian family, education is viewed as the only means of upward socioeconomic mobility. This philosophy is deeply rooted in the core of the society, whose political leaders speak so passionately of "democracy through education." In practically every country in the West Indies, there are role models of poor citizens who became political leaders after attaining advanced education. Calypsonians, such as the Mighty Sparrow and other artists, expound the value of education in their songs—"Children, go to school and learn well. Otherwise later on you will catch real hell." Education is emphasized in every facet of the society, and everyone believes there is no limit on upward mobility for the person who is highly educated. As the West Indian citizen understands it, a person's horizons are not limited by race or religion, but by a lack of education. And the major limitation is a country's inability, because of economic factors, to educate all its citizens. There are not enough public high schools in the larger countries to accommodate all potential students (as discussed in Chapter 2). In the smaller countries, where the potential student body is much smaller, all are able to attend high school. There are some private schools throughout the West Indies, but only the affluent can afford to educate their children privately. In the West Indian culture, university education is not a prerequisite for employment—many persons who have risen through the ranks to become top civil servants have held only high school certificates. This means that those who have university degrees receive the best appointments and more lucrative salaries.

Other factors besides the shortage of schools limit educational opportunities for West Indian children. Climate is one such factor. During the rainy season, which lasts from June to December, floods sometimes block roads and prevent children from attending school regularly. Even more devastating are the occasional hurricanes: In 1988 and 1989, Hurricanes Gilbert and Hugo, respectively, hit several West Indian islands (notably Jamaica, St. Kitts and Nevis, Montserrat, Antigua, and St. Croix). Another factor that can disrupt schooling is the continuing political unrest characteristic of several West Indian nations, to say nothing of events such as the U.S. invasion of Grenada in 1983. (Chapter 11 has more to say about the educational and psychological effects of natural disaster and political strife on West Indian children.) Finally, familial economic hardship can pose a barrier to education, especially in rural areas. Children may have to help their families farm the land, and girls sometimes have to help their mothers in the home and to care for younger siblings.

Because of the paucity of funds for schools, the typical classroom in the West Indies has a rather bland appearance. For the most part, there are chairs, desks, a chalkboard, and chalk, but visual aids are in short supply. Equipment in science laboratories is very limited at the elementary level and relatively limited at the high school level, particularly in rural areas. Children even share textbooks and maps. Thus the average West Indian child is less exposed to hands-on, practical types of experiences. Educators responsible for the university entrance examination have, however, begun to stress the need to remedy this for high school students.

Whereas the learning experiences of U.S. students tend to be action-oriented (learning by doing) and visual, those of West Indian students are more auditory and teacher-oriented. Students are expected to be attentive to their teachers' instruction all day, even though it is often merely a board that separates one class from another. Thus it is quite possible for students to hear what is going on in another classroom. This may help explain why the average West Indian student, upon entry into the U.S. school system, is often described as being very quiet in the classroom. To such a student, the classroom is a place to listen and pay attention. And when these students are bombarded with visual aids, with little auditory stimulation, they often experience difficulty. West Indian children may appear to be less academically motivated because of this difference in instructional patterns.

Chapter 11 discusses the effect of different learning styles on retention and recall; it also examines the effect of language (West Indian Creole) on an immigrant child's ability to integrate into the education system. Students who do not get into academically oriented high schools generally learn a trade at a worksite or go to a vocational school, where only about 20% of the curriculum is academic. Thus when these children enter the U.S. school system at age 14, they have not been educated in the academic sense for about two years. Families tend not to be receptive to vocational schools, perceiving them as an inferior alternative to traditional academic education. Thus West Indian parents push their children to take every opportunity to get an education when they come to the United States. As far as West Indian parents are concerned, the onus of achieving is on the students, not on a system construed by some to be racist (see Chapter 8).

Likewise, West Indian Americans place the onus on adults to work as many jobs as necessary to provide for family members—both in the United States and in their native lands. Because the economies of the West Indies are not flourishing and because unemployment there is relatively high, it is very rare that anyone is able to hold two jobs. The tendency of many West Indian Americans to work two jobs does not reflect a common practice in the islands.

In the West Indies, success is defined by family values and educational attainment. The hard work displayed by West Indian Americans is a direct result of the immigrants' philosophy of making use of every opportunity while it lasts.

To West Indian Americans, success is measured by one's educational level, material possessions, ability to travel (be it home to the West Indies or elsewhere), and ability to entertain friends. Owning a house (no matter how small) is part of their cultural upbringing; people simply do not rent houses as others do in the United States. The intense desire of West Indians to own their own homes is quite in keeping with their cultural mores. Beyond the house, West Indian Americans have learned, via the television and other media, to endorse the North American definition of success, which includes materialism. Thus the family/education-oriented definition of success that prevails in the West Indies takes second place to the North American definition. The ultimate result is that parents are not as available to their children as they were in their native lands. Emotional support and "quality time" are minimal in comparison to the support afforded to these children back home. Thus when behavioral problems arise with their children, the parents experience frustration and helplessness, claiming passionately, "We have given our children everything—a home, clothes, money, an education." What they fail to realize is that a materialistic definition of success can have negative influences. Chapters 11 and 12 examine the effect of the absent parent on the immigrant child.

WORK PATTERN IN THE WEST INDIES

In the West Indies, most people are employed as civil servants or in the areas of tourism or agriculture. Private industries are mainly involved in trade and commerce, such as the retail industry, shipping, and construction. The government is heavily involved in the tourist industry. Since only a minority of the population is self-employed, most people are affected when the countries are in an economic depression. The East Indians in Trinidad and Guyana tend to be self-employed in small businesses and agriculture. This is probably why they are doing better than most other groups today, in spite of the economic crisis in the West Indies. Chapter 5 discusses the East Indians in more detail.

This employment pattern highlights culturally based differences that are important for understanding West Indian immigrants. It explains, for example, why West Indian immigrants tend to feel more comfortable working for the government in secure, salaried jobs. Unlike the Chinese and East Indians, who tend to be self-employed in small businesses, people of African background in the West Indies generally assume government positions upon completion of school. In the United States, Canada, and Britain as well, they settle into government jobs for the most part. The few who are self-employed live with the continued fear that anything can happen at any time; as they see it, this justifies their need to work long hours even at the expense of their families.

CHAPTER 5

Racism

"Racism does not exist in the West Indies." This is the statement generally made by West Indian Americans when faced with the question of racism. Interestingly, of the people in the West Indies who responded to the West Indian Attitude Survey (Appendix V), approximately 86% said there are racial problems in the West Indies, even though they recognized that these problems were less severe than in the United States, Canada, or Great Britain. Fewer West Indian immigrants (60%), when given the Immigrant Attitude Survey (Appendix IV), whether in the United States, Canada, or Britain, felt that racial problems existed in the West Indies. It seems that once they migrate, West Indian immigrants experience a more intense form of racism that makes them trivialize the reality of racism in the West Indies.

I (Gopaul-McNicol, 1986, 1988) used black and white dolls to examine racial identification and racial preference in 144 preschool children from Trinidad and Tobago. Later, 302 preschool children were tested throughout several West Indian islands—Jamaica, Trinidad and Tobago, Barbados, and Grenada. As in a much earlier study (Clark & Clark, 1947), a substantial majority of the children aged 3 to 6 showed a preference for the white doll and identified with the white doll. Even most of the dark-skinned black children chose the white doll as their look-alike and as being the nice doll. Likewise, most of the black children chose the black doll as "looking bad." In the West Indies, social class did not affect racial preference; the socioeconomic status of children made no significant difference in their doll preference. What was particularly disturbing were the spontaneous remarks made by the children, such as "I don't like being black" and "I will be rich if I am like the white doll."

33

The issue, of course, is why these children made such comments and showed such a strong white preference. It is likely that they were reflecting the prevailing social attitude in the West Indies—that to be powerful, beautiful, or economically successful, one ought to be white or light-skinned. Phillips (1976) reported a study conducted by Miller (1967), who examined self-concept and color-related features in Jamaican children. The report showed that the most frequent concerns were skin color, hair, and the shape of the nose and lips. It was found that the girls of African heritage longed for long, straight hair like that of the white, Chinese, and East Indian children. Phillips (1976) noted that the "dissatisfaction with color appeared only among the brown, dark and black" (p. 31). An explicit picture of the ideal self was given by the children in their description of the handsome boy. "Good looking" meant "blue or pretty eyes, a straight nose, a small mouth, clear complexion, straight or wavy hair" (Phillips, 1976, p. 45). Young and Bagley (1979) reported similar findings.

It is possible that a feeling of white supremacy, despite the many black leaders throughout the West Indies, is a legacy of the British colonial education system. The school curriculum gives little attention to the contributions of West Indian leaders both in the West Indies and abroad. For example, it is disturbing to note that a chapter on drugs in a major English textbook uses a picture of a black man, while a picture of a Caucasian man is used in a discussion of science. Thus, although the standard textbooks do not purposely humiliate any of the groups that comprise the population, racist stereotypes prevail to this day. This white bias subtly permeates every facet of these societies; people feel they have had a better education if they were educated in Great Britain as opposed to the West Indies or the United States. Parents speak with great pride of their children studying in Britain, regardless of the ranking of the schools. In spite of the continued oppression of West Indians in Britain and the continued contempt the British government has for the West Indies (see Chapter 9), West Indians continue to credit the British for "giving us a good education" (an education that never taught its people racial self-identification and cultural pride). If children see the development of the West Indies solely as a result of European or American influences, this may deprive them of the pride that comes from being an integral part of the West Indies.

Another possible explanation for the white preference is the impact of the media. The most important purveyor of contemporary culture is probably the television, and this medium is predominantly American. The same shows that are shown in America are shown in the West Indies, with the same white bias.

Although one is able to purchase black dolls in the West Indies, most of the children I surveyed (Gopaul-McNicol, 1986, 1988) had only white dolls at home, suggesting that parents believe white dolls are better to play with. Children implicitly incorporate the attitudes of their parents and of society into their value systems.

Yet another reason for the belief that being white is preferable is that this view simply reflects prevailing economic realities. It was only after the West Indian black power movement of the 1970s (see Chapter 7) that dark-skinned people were seriously considered for employment in banks and as flight attendants—jobs that had usually been given to whites or mulattos. Although this situation is not as flagrant today, 73% of the individuals residing in the West Indies who responded to the West Indian Attitude Survey believe that the lighter one is, the better are one's chances for upward social mobility. Educational success is a necessary, but not sufficient, requirement for upward mobility by a black person.

IS IT CLASS OR RACE?

While racism exists in the West Indies, the fact that people of African ancestry make up 80% to 90% of the population in most areas (except in Trinidad and Guyana, where East Indians comprise about 41%) makes the African West Indian less threatened by outside influences, and this is probably why West Indian political leaders are mainly of African heritage. However, whites on the islands are concentrated in the higher-priced and more desirable residential areas, indicating that ethnic differences are often reinforced by economics. It is indisputable that the most affluent people in the West Indies are the European or American whites, with few blacks and some mulattos being considered very wealthy. This suggests that European standards still prevail, in spite of the political independence of many of the islands. It can be argued that those who have money—those who control the media and the multinational lending agencies—are the ones who are really in power and the ones who dictate policies in the region.

The reason racism is so often difficult for many West Indians to articulate is that "color and class interweave to such an extent that it is nearly impossible and in any case impractical, to separate each from the other" (Phillips, 1976, p. 27). This claim can be further empirically supported if one looks at the social structure. Kerr (1952), Hendriques (1953), Miller (1967), and De Albuquerque (1989) all contend that the lighter-skinned people, including the Chinese, tend to belong to the upper social class, while people of darker skin color tend to belong to the lower class. There is a very small middle class, made up of mulattos or blacks, while the large lower class is predominantly black with a few mulattos (Phillips, 1976). The fact that whites, who number less than 5% of the population, completely dominate the upper class, while the blacks dominate the lower and middle classes seems to confirm that ethnic differences are reinforced by socioeconomic differences. To some people, the medium of social economics seems to be a rather roundabout approach to racial inequalities. Of course, one can argue that the middle class has political power. However "political power minus economic power" leaves people "still politically paralyzed before their former masters. They are political nouveaux-riches" (Ambursley & Cohen, 1983, p. 9). Thus in the West Indies class and color are indeed interwoven, probably because "the long years of subjugation by European powers have made ethnicity an important foci of the class struggle" (Ambursley & Cohen, 1983, p. 5).

RACISM IN TRINIDAD AND GUYANA—AFRICANS VERSUS EAST INDIANS

After the African slave trade had ended, there was a need to maintain the plantation system in order to keep whites supreme (Rodney, 1983) in the West Indian colonies. This led to East Indian immigration to the West Indies. East Indians from Calcutta were brought into Georgetown, Guyana, and later Trinidad. However, the agents of the Anti-Slavery Society told tales of gross ill-treatment of the East Indians, claiming that "East Indian immigration is merely another form of slavery" (Daniel, 1952, Vol. 3, p. 269). So loud was the cry that a ban was placed on East Indian immigration. Nevertheless, East Indians continued to migrate to these two countries not as indentured servants but in search of work, because "the British commercial, military, and political parties destroyed the life and culture of 19th century India" (Rodney, 1983, p. 26). Today, East Indians make up about 41% of the population in Trinidad and Guyana.

When the East Indians first arrived, they lived rather humbly, which enabled them to accumulate money. For the most part today, they live in fine houses, educate their children, and are entrepreneurial. Because of their expanding businesses and their understanding of the social value of money, many of them have acquired social prominence and status. It is remarkable that in large measure those of East Indian descent born in the West Indies are still seen as "foreigners" by many of the West Indians of African descent in Trinidad and Guyana. Some people feel that this sentiment was corroborated by a cricket match in 1971, when a team from India played against a team from the West Indies. Apparently, the passionate support that those of East Indian descent in Trinidad gave to the cricketers from India led to the accusation that "they are not really West Indians." This attitude still prevails to some extent.

It seems that several institutions—the plantation, the church, and the school—may all have contributed to the East Indian–African antagonism, which may have its roots in cultural and economic forces. In addition, a major contributing factor was the fear that if the East Indian children attended school, they would be forced to convert to Christianity and give up their Hindi language, since Christianity was the focus in the schools at that time. Therefore, as late as 1911, 97% of the East Indian-born population of Trinidad was illiterate (Bereton, 1985). This is where the connection with Canada came into play for the East Indians of Trinidad and Guyana. Canadian missionaries established a college for training Canadian mission teachers. They also established a network of elementary and secondary schools that began around 1930 to educate East Indian children, using the Hindi language if the need arose. Today, compulsory education exists for all children. All children are taught in English and many people of East Indian descent have accepted Christianity, but many others have maintained their Hindu or Muslim faith. In spite of the endeavors to temper race relations, many politicians have used this issue for their own political gain. In fact, the bitter feelings are so profound that a separatist National Indesh Freedom Party was formed in Canada, where most of the East Indian immigrants from Trinidad and Guyana tend to migrate. This party "aims to establish a separate state within the boundaries of Trinidad, because of the years of suppression of the basic human rights of the East Indian population in Trinidad" (Regional Newspaper for the North Eastern Caribbean, 1991, p. 2). Thus racism or conflict in the form of Africans versus East Indians (which began at the end of the nineteenth century), with whites in support of one group or the other at different times, depending on circumstances, exists today in Trinidad and Guyana.

THE MEANING OF "BLACK" IN THE WEST INDIES AND ITS IMPLICATION ON ACCULTURATION AFTER MIGRATION

It is the dominant "mother country" that has defined who is black and who is white. To Britain, "if you are not White, then you are Black" (Rodney, 1983, p. 16). However, it is evident that the West Indian situation is highly complex, with a variety of racial mixtures. Therefore one cannot merely rely on the European or American definition of "black" and "white," but must look to how people perceive themselves and one another. Although the vast majority of West Indian people are by European definition "black," because they are either African or East Indian, many people do not think of themselves in color terminologies. To this day, "Negro" is still used by many to describe Africans and "Indian" is used to describe East Indians. Thus when the black power movement began in the early 1970s, the East Indians felt that this movement was being aimed at them, in spite of the fact that they experienced the same racial contempt from whites as did those of African descent. It is felt that the East Indians in the West Indies remain concerned that espousing a West Indian identity would in effect deny expression of their own culture and history, since they comprise a relatively small percentage of the population in the West Indies as a whole.

The mulattos, the West Indian light-skinned persons of European and African descent, are characterized by ambivalence—they are termed "West Indian whites." Some have identified with the black masses; others have not. The Chinese West Indians, on the other hand, see themselves as "bastions of the white West Indian social structure" (Rodney, 1983, p. 28). The Syrians, Europeans, and Jews all consider themselves white.

Racial self-perception plays an important role in the overall adjustment of immigrants of color from the West Indies. Those who perceived themselves as black before they migrated tend to adjust more easily with respect to the European or American definition of "black." Those who perceived themselves as white, mixed, or East Indian usually go through a period of denial when they are termed "black" by the European or American society. The WICAB (Appendix II), under the heading "Racial Attitude," helps in determining the level of difficulty (or lack thereof) that West Indians experience with respect to racial adjustment upon migration.

CHAPTER 6

Notable Differences Among the Islands

While the previous chapters have given a general overview of West Indian immigrants, it is important to note when working with West Indian families that among West Indians, as among African Americans, there is diversity. Since there is a potential for stereotyping in the ethnicity literature, I am particularly concerned that interisland differences—a sensitive issue for West Indians themselves—not be overlooked. Although it is beyond the scope of this book to provide a detailed analysis of these differences, too much cultural generalization can be harmful. The structural formations outlined thus far in this book represent the West Indian islands accurately. There are some major differences, however, that must be mentioned.

There is a strong movement toward integration among the eastern Caribbean islands (St. Kitts and Nevis, Antigua and Barbuda, Montserrat, Grenada, St. Vincent and the Grenadines, St. Lucia); these islands share the same currency, making trade and sociopolitical relations easier among them. In addition, Trinidad and Tobago, St. Vincent, and Grenada are linked by a strong sociopolitical and economic bond because of the historical movement of population among these countries. This helps explain the social interdependence and to some extent the shared loyalties of Trinidadians, Grenadians, and Vincentians in the United States.

Chapter 5 has briefly discussed the racial differences in Trinidad and Guyana, and the political link between the East Indians in Trinidad and Guyana. In Guyana there are major production problems in the domestic economy, in spite of its vast amount of land (all of the West Indian islands could fit into Guyana, which is bigger than England). Reviving the Guyanese economy will require massive financial inflows from foreign countries. Confidence has to be restored in its people in order to regain the respect of its regional partners and other countries. In addition, the breakdown of the education system and emigration have denuded this society of its educated and trained human resources. Like those of Haiti, the special circumstances of Guyana deserve careful study and research. However, this is beyond the scope of this chapter.

The West Indian countries are very small. Guyana, the largest, has an area of 83,000 square miles. Next come the Bahamas and Jamaica, with 5,400 and 4,411 square miles, respectively. With the exception of Trinidad and Tobago, which combined make up 1,980 square miles, the remaining islands range from 33 square miles (Montserrat) to 305 square miles (Dominica). The populations are also small, ranging from approximately 13,000 in Montserrat to 2.2 million in Jamaica. (The size of Jamaica's population, relative to that of other islands, helps explain why there are more Jamaicans than other islanders in the United States, Britain, and Canada.) Together, the West Indian countries have a population of about 6 million.

Since Jamaica lies on the outer periphery of the West Indies, it is the island least integrated with the others. Its major links are sports, Rastafarianism, an intellectual elite, and CARICOM. This chapter will briefly address the distinct sociopolitical differences of Jamaican culture, since it differs in certain aspects from West Indian culture as discussed thus far, and since so many West Indian immigrants in the United States, Britain, and Canada are Jamaicans.

Relative to the other islanders, the Jamaican people tend to be distinctly assertive. I was told by a descendant of a former slave of the Maroon tribe—a statement I was unable to corroborate in my literature search—that during the transporting of slaves from Africa to the West Indies, Jamaica was the first stop along the way. Here the more rebellious and aggressive slaves were dropped off, since they had created problems on the journey. Some of these slaves later came to be known as the Maroons—the word comes from the Spanish word *cimarron*, which means "wild, unruly." Escaped slaves used to join the Maroons, who remained a formidable threat to the development of the colony's plantation system. The colonists fought desperately to remove the Maroons, whom they saw as a menace. Although the Maroons were never really completely defeated, they lost many men and faced starvation. Thus in the 1730s, when the governor of the island offered to sign a treaty guaranteeing the Maroons ownership of a specific area of land in the Cockpit County, the Maroons' leader, Cudjoe, agreed. This is very significant in understanding Jamaican immigrants and even the Rastafarian culture. Wherever they have migrated, Jamaicans are viewed as the ones least tolerant of discrimination. The history of their forebears sheds some light on the reasons for their assertiveness. Of course, because of their numerical preponderance, Jamaicans are able to maintain their cultural identification more easily than any of the other islanders. Their reggae music has reached around the world, and for many years, Americans would ask "whether Trinidad is in Jamaica."

A noted difference in the Jamaican culture is the strength and independence of many of the women, in comparison to the women of other islands. This can be attributed to the difficulty the men experienced in obtaining employment within their own communities, requiring them to work far away from home (the island is relatively large); in some cases they came home only on weekends. Thus the women were responsible not only for the home and child care, but for helping with production of crops and administrative matters. This might explain why there are more single mothers among Jamaicans than among the other islanders. Of course, since Jamaica has had the longest history of migration to the United States, Britain, and Canada, the culture of these countries may also have had a significant impact on the attitudes of Jamaicans.

Jamaica is beset with problems of overpopulation, poverty, and limited academic educational opportunities for all children; as discussed in Chapters 2 and 4, approximately 75% of children do not receive the traditonal academic high school education (a higher percentage than in all other West Indian islands). This is probably why most of the West Indian children who are experiencing educational difficulties in Britain, the United States, and Canada are of Jamaican background. At Multicultural Educational and Psychological Services P.C., 70% of the West Indian families who are referred by the schools for educational and psychological services are of Jamaican background. Of even greater concern is a recent report from the New York State Department of Correctional Services (Clarke, 1991) indicating that from April 1, 1985, to December 31, 1991, while the number of inmates born in the United States increased by 54%, the number of foreign-born inmates increased by 148%. Approximately two-thirds of the foreign-born inmates originally came from the Dominican Republic, Colombia, Cuba, or Jamaica, with Jamaica ranking second behind the Dominican Republic. Of course, the high number of Jamaican inmates could be due to the fact that Jamaicans are the second-largest group of immigrants in New York City (New York City

Department of Planning, 1985). Moreover, it was found that only 4% of the foreign-born inmates were naturalized citizens; two-fifths were in the United States illegally, and the status of the others was described as "tenuous at best" (Clarke, 1991, p. 1).

It is important to note that there are ingroup differences in Jamaica, such as those between a Jamaican from an urban center (such as Kingston) and one from a rural area. Those from urban areas are more exposed to modern Western culture and are therefore more influenced by the Western mode of living. Cultural adjustment tends to be less traumatic for them.

The Rastafarian movement, which originated in Jamaica, is a culture of its own. The next chapter discusses this movement in detail.

CHAPTER 7

Rastafarian/Rastafari Culture

One cannot discuss the West Indian people without exploring the Rastafarian/Rastafari culture, since this movement has had a profound impact on West Indian society, especially that of Jamaica.

WHAT IS A RASTA?

The Rastafarian/Rastafari movement came to world consciousness via Jamaica. It first began as a "religious counteraction to the imperialistic outcomes of Eurocentric Christendom" (Semaj, 1979, p. 8). As stated by Rogers (1975a), Rastafarians, otherwise known as Rastafari or Rastas, stress positive change by such means as the following:

1. Awareness by black people of their African heritage.
2. Recognition of the former emperor of Ethiopia, Haile Selassie, as the black reincarnated Christ.
3. Repatriation to Ethiopia/Africa, the true home of all blacks.
4. The apocalyptic fall of Jamaica as Babylon, the corrupt world of the white man.

THE HISTORY OF THE RASTAFARI MOVEMENT

In 1927 the black leader Marcus Garvey returned from the United States to his homeland, Jamaica. Garvey is said to have told the

Jamaican people to "look to Africa when a Black king shall be crowned, for the day of deliverance is near" (Gordon, 1960, p. 5). Following Garvey, the Rastas contend that black persons who have made little attempt to redefine or recreate their African culture are an impediment in the struggle for liberation of African people. Rastas have been identified as having a different appearance, lifestyle, linguistic usage, religion, and overall attitude. They have attempted to reverse the syndrome "the Black man has nothing and has no chance of getting anything" (Rogers, 1975a, p. 12). Broadly speaking, the Rastas' doctrines are radical because they reject the "black masses" category and define themselves as separate from the wider Jamaican society. They constantly reaffirm their Africanness and speak out against the economic oppression of black people. They emphasize that they will deal only with their brethren on their terms, not those "handed down from plantation society" (Rogers, 1975a, p. 12). They contend that when Jamaica became independent in 1962, the power was merely transferred from the British to the brown and white elite.

Semaj (1979) has explained that the Rastafari movement after Garvey's death in 1940 evolved in three phases:

1. The 1940s through the 1960s saw the attempted destruction of the Rastafari movement by such labels as "religious fanatics," "nuisances," and "an embarrassment to the Jamaican people." At that time the British and then the Jamaican government attempted (by degrading the movement) to bring the Rastas to their senses with respect to repatriation to Africa.

2. The years 1971 to 1981 saw the expansion of the concept of the Rastafari at home and abroad. Two people were closely associated with this phase: Michael Manley, whose People's National Party provided a political context for the expression of things African and black, and Bob Marley, who espoused Rastafarian doctrines in his music. During this phase, even the uptown people's children were "going dread."

3. In 1980 Manley was removed from office in Jamaica, resulting in a dramatic change in the country's policies. Then Bob Marley died in 1981. These events meant the collapse of the context that had partially facilitated expansion and acceptance of Rastafarianism.

Today the Rastafari movement has spread around the world—in particular, the West Indies, the United States, Great Britain, and Canada. It is considered an important, politically potent organizing concept for African people, particularly youths. Young people use this movement to speak out against white oppression, to foster a black identity, and to develop a unique linguistic style. Some teachers say that some students, particularly boys, use the Rastafari language as a form of opposition to school authorities and as a way of excluding them from their conversations. The Rasta students who participated in the Immigrant Attitude Survey (Appendix IV) said that via the Rastafari culture they are able to achieve their own political and social space in a school environment they perceive as hostile and foreign.

ASPECTS OF RASTAFARI CULTURE

Appearance

"Dreadlocks," or "the crown of glory," are primarily what set the Rastas apart from others in society. According to Rasta doctrines, this practice of allowing the hair to grow and then plaiting it (which forms the locks) dates back to the Old Testament, "when the Lord declared to his children that whosoever shall follow me shall never take scissors to his hair, nor razor to his face." Historically, this was a common practice among Ethiopian warriors. The Rasta women do not straighten their hair.

The treatment of the hair is the most obvious source of dispute among the Rastas. There are three categories:

1. The locksmen, whose hair is matted, plaited, and never cut. The beard is never cut either.
2. The beardsmen, who grow the hair and beard but may occasionally trim them. They do not plait the hair.
3. The baldheads, or clean-faced men who look like ordinary Jamaicans except for the "heavenly" colored scarf they wear; in some cases, they wear the beard. The baldheads tend to be government-employed. Although they do not openly declare themselves to be brethren, they are deeply sensitive and sympathetic to the Rastafari doctrines and movement. Because they believe that the Jamaican government is still hostile and discriminatory toward Rastas, they take a different view regarding their appearance.

Rastas in the first two categories wear moustaches as well. In general, because they have difficulty obtaining government or other employment, they have small businesses of their own. They regard themselves as the ones who have endured the most suffering for their race and religion.

Rastas are also known for their "heavenly" colors—gold, green, and red, which are the colors of Ethiopia. Gold signifies the riches of the Ethiopian soil; green, peace and forgiveness; and red, judgment upon the wicked rulers of Babylon and the salvation of all black people around the world.

Food

The Rastas eat neither pork nor shellfish. They claim that hogs are unclean, the scavengers of the earth, and that shellfish (such as crab, shrimp, and lobster) are the scavengers of the sea. They prefer to eat smaller fish rather than larger ones, such as kingfish or barracuda, because the latter are cannibalistic. They also prefer "ital foods"—that is, foods that are organically grown and chemically untreated. Rastas tend to avoid strong liquor, such as rum, because they believe that consuming alcohol is harmful to the mind and body. They also contend that white people oppress black people via alcohol.

Family

Rastafarian males have strong patriarchal tendencies and tend to make kind, gentle, and responsible fathers (De Albuquerque, 1979). Children are usually seen with their fathers in the Rasta camps because the Rastas believe that children complement their lives. Rastas usually want their children (especially boys) to live with them so that they can be raised with an understanding of their African heritage. Their love for children is widely acknowledged. They tend to adopt children and make great sacrifices to take care of them. A woman is treated with great respect and is referred to as a "queen." Rasta males are accorded much deference in their society. Therefore major conflicts tend to arise when they migrate to the United States, Britain, and Canada, where women assume positions of leadership and are often the chief breadwinners (see Chapters 12 and 14).

Education and Work Values

Rastafarians believe strongly in formal education. They encourage youths to attend school, in spite of their belief that the education system helps to colonialize and "de-Africanize" black children. They have also emphasized an individualized pedagogy—"each one teach one." Some Rastas send their children to private schools, even if they have to pay, because they fear that their children will be mocked because of their dreadlocks and beliefs in the public schools.

Many Rastas refuse to work for the government because of its

"Babylonian attitudes," instead working for themselves as fishermen, farmers, or skilled craftsmen. Whether self-employed or working for wages, Rastas tend to be conscientious workers. They also help support their unskilled brethren who are unemployed. Unemployment is one of the major problems facing Rastas. This is attributable partly to discrimination based on appearance, partly to the high unemployment rate throughout the society, and possibly partly to the attraction of the movement for the unemployed.

Art

Rastafarian artists range from poets to sculptors. The Akete drums are played by many of the brethren. Performing or listening to music, such as reggae, is a form of entertainment typical of the Jamaican people.

Religion

Rastas, unlike many in the wider West Indian society, do not believe in obeah (a form of witchcraft, discussed in more detail in Chapters 11 and 12) or magic; they view them as nonsense. Their religious tradition is anthropomorphic; they believe in God, but believe He is black and has their African features. The Rastafari have taken a culturally and politically revolutionary step in asserting that God reflects their own image—one that some see as important in the struggle of the African people for self-respect. The religious orthodoxy of the Rastas is, however, on the decline among the young people. This could be attributed to the failure of prophecy. Many Rastas have turned toward more fundamental churches and toward Christianity. Some have moved from a religious ideology to a political one, such as socialism; however, with the fall of communism around the world, there is less socialist sentiment. Thus the Rastas who have maintained their religious orthodoxy are being isolated more and more from society, in spite of their popularity in Jamaica.

DISCRIMINATION AND THE RASTAS

Throughout the Caribbean, the United States, Great Britain, and Canada, the Rastafari have largely been seen in the context of reggae music, the dreadlocks, and unfounded propaganda that Rastas are violent.

In 1989, I was in line at the Barbados airport waiting to be checked in. There was a Rastafarian in line ahead of me. No one in front of him encountered any difficulty, so the line was moving along well. The Rasta, however, underwent an intense verbal search, being questioned about his intent, political belief, whether he was carrying drugs, and so forth. This, to me, was harassment, so I asked to speak to a supervisor. The supervisor offered no explanation for this persecution, but rather asked about my relationship to this man. The superiors were appalled that a woman of my educational status, who knew nothing of this man, would come to his defense so passionately. In any event, the man (whom I later came to know was a teacher) was finally permitted to board the plane. After interviewing many Rastas in the West Indies, United States, and England, I realize that they encounter such reactions practically every day of their lives. In the British Virgin Islands, the Prohibited Persons Act, which went into effect in 1980, states that all Rastas are barred from entering the country unless they are questioned and undergo a strip search. Although there are no such laws in the other Caribbean islands, on a daily basis Rastas experience excessive questioning, disrespect, and outright discrimination.

CRIME AND THE RASTAS

In 1985 the intelligence division of the New York City Police Department prepared a report on Rastas. The strategic analysis revealed that only a small portion of the total Rastafarian community is involved in crime and that "all Rastas are not criminals." What is of particular concern is that many people who present themselves as Rastas are imposters who simply use the Rasta appearance to cover up their criminal activity. They, too, know that the Rastas are discriminated against and are confident that the legal system will believe the Rastas to be the criminals.

Since the Rastafari doctrine is considered by the wider society as radical in that it is against the oppression of blacks, there are some who have linked the movement to Marxism. This is not the case. The movement has been infiltrated by a number of criminals, but these people are basically individualists who have little ideological influence. The true Rastafarian brethren call these criminals "rudeboys." It is this group within the Rastafarian movement that seems to be drawing attention in United States, Canada, and Britain. A "true Rasta is a law abiding proud individual, who has total commitment to the Rastafarian religion" (New York City Police Department, 1985, p. 12). Rastas do not condone acts of violence. The report says that true Rastas are hardworking and "fear the criminal elements of their cult" (New

York City Police Department, 1985, p. 39). However, since they believe in reincarnation and do not fear death, they will defend themselves if they are attacked. For the most part, these are relatively peaceful, religious people who have a strong sense of racial identification. Their intent is to educate themselves, their children, and their brethren about Africa and the black man. Neither violence nor criminal activity is condoned. "In many ways Rasta communities offer refuge to ghetto youth weary of the violence of West Kingston" (De Albuquerque, 1979, p. 25).

DRUGS AND THE RASTAS

Their abstention from alcohol, noted above, sets the Rastas apart from the wider society (De Albuquerque, 1979). The use of marijuana (ganja) is accorded religious significance; it is seen as "a gift of God, who enjoined one to smoke it in Genesis 8, Psalms 18 and Revelations 22" (Gordon, 1960, p. 22). Some brethren have nothing to do with ganja, while others use it for therapeutic reasons, such as supposedly keeping away illnesses. They use the marijuana herb as tea in the morning; smoke it in a ritual manner, passing it from one person to the next; and use it as medicine when ill. When I visited the Rasta camps in Jamaica and observed the children drinking marijuana tea for breakfast, I realized that the Rastas do not think that marijuana is harmful. For them, it is an integral part of their daily living pattern. It is referred to as "the wisdom weed" or "the holy herb" and is considered one of the best ways to relax and be in union with God. If it is not illegal to drink rum, they ask, why is it illegal to smoke ganja? Of course, the Rastas are concerned that drug dealers exploit their religious beliefs in order to protect the trade in narcotics. They believe that the government and the media have portrayed the Rastas as substance abusers, when they (drug dealers) have been beneficiaries of the narcotics trade. If the Rastas are behind drug trafficking, they ask, why are they not as affluent as drug lords normally are?

POLITICS AND THE RASTAS: PAST AND FUTURE

Anita Waters (1984) has brought to the forefront the use of the Rastas in Jamaican politics. To a large extent, she feels that the electoral success of the People's National Party in 1972 and the Jamaica Labor Party in 1980 resulted from each party's ability to reflect and appropriate Rastafarian music and symbols in relation to lower-class protest. At that time the Rastas were seen as the "conscience of society" (with Bob Marley as their spokesman), and thus the movement was germane to politics.

While it was possible to use the Rastafarian movement in the 1970s and 1980s in politics, the 1990s seem to be different. The Rastafarian utopian–messianic beliefs, while not completely on the fringes of society, clearly do not have as much influence as in the prior two decades; however, they are still popular among leftist academics and politicians. No one will denounce the movement outright for fear of being labeled an imperialist. The strategy is thus to identify, recognize, and be sensitive to the movement publicly, while privately condemning it as a barrier to the construction of a true capitalist Jamaica.

The Rastafarians in Jamaica will probably function as two subgroups in the future. One group (the Ethiopian messianic type) will remain uncompromising in their ideals and will continue to live on the fringes of society. A second group (probably the larger group), comprised of the working class, will be less committed to the religious ideology and more concerned with the cultural or even political aspects of the movement. This group will tend to act as a buffer between the Rastas who are unemployed and the critics of the movement. The Rastas must either help to chart a course for Jamaica or be less critical of government policies. An alliance between the two Rasta groups is needed, because a "laissez-faire" attitude has existed since the death of Bob Marley. What is also needed is a serious Rasta intelligentsia—that is, those who will extrapolate or transform the oral to the written, and those who will be more economically and politically assertive. The Rastafari movement can indeed continue to be a vehicle for the laboring class to express their feelings, their African ancestry, and the rendition of God in their own image.

CHAPTER 8

Differences Between African Americans and African West Indian Americans

In politics, in the professional litera-
ture, and in education, little distinction is made among black cultural
subgroups. Thus the black West Indian immigrant is viewed in the
same manner as the black who was born and raised in the United
States. Boyd-Franklin (1989) clearly emphasizes that "Black West
Indians and their immigration patterns to the United States [are] an
area worthy of careful study in the research and clinical literature" (p.
7). However, several authors who have written on the black family or
raising black children have erroneously suggested that the same
techniques can be applied in working with West Indian blacks.
Approaching all blacks in the United States as a monolithic group
presents problems for West Indian immigrants, whose family structure
and ethnic identification are different, given their different cultural
experiences. When therapists approach therapy with black West
Indian immigrants in very much the same manner as they approach
therapy with African Americans—as they often do—the result is client
mistrust of the therapeutic process, communication difficulties, and
ultimately therapeutic resistance.

Obviously, American and West Indian blacks share a common
African heritage; some slaves were sent to the West Indies and others
to the United States. But the numerical preponderance of blacks in the

West Indies (approximately 82% of the total population is black) has allowed black West Indians to hold on to their African culture more than blacks in America, who are and always have been a distinct minority. This difference is compounded by the reality that West Indian migration to the United States was and remains voluntary. Herein lies the fundamental difference between black Americans and black West Indian Americans. West Indian immigrants feel that they left their ghost of slavery behind when they migrated voluntarily to the United States for a better life. And unlike black Americans, who feel disconnected from their African roots, black West Indians attempt to maintain a cultural identification with their native islands. They continue to view themselves as immigrants and to assert their identity in order to distinguish themselves from black Americans. They fill their neighborhoods with cultural expressions that pay tribute to their island heritage.

In the United States, the legacy of slavery lives on in the hearts and minds of the African American, primarily because the existence of the slave society depended on the perpetual subjugation of the African. Impassable barriers between the races were upheld by institutional racism in the United States. By contrast, in the West Indies the brutality of racism was softened and masked by the concept of "social color, whereby a person's particular classification in the total scheme was determined not always so much by skin color, but by other criteria [such] as education, social position and wealth" (Lewis, 1983). Thus, while money merely talks in the United States, in the West Indies money both talks and whitens. Even so, prejudice in the West Indies, masked or subtle as it may be at times, cannot be excused.

CONTRIBUTIONS OF WEST INDIANS IN THE UNITED STATES

From their first entry into the United States, West Indians have contributed to the upward mobility and liberation of all those of African descent. In politics, entertainment, sports, and business, the West Indian contribution has been significant.

In politics, the roster of distinguished West Indian immigrants includes Alexander Hamilton of Nevis, who was Washington's chief of staff, an architect of the Constitution, and the first secretary of the treasury. In the late 1700s, Jean Baptiste Pointe DuSable, a native of Haiti, founded the trading post on the southwest tip of Lake Michigan that later grew into Chicago. In the 1920s, Marcus Garvey, originally from Jamaica, in his Pan-Africanist movement envisioned the creation of an independent black government in Africa; he also formed the

Universal Negro Improvement Association, an organization with as many as 6 million members worldwide, whose focus was on uniting blacks internationally. Historically, it was the first and largest mass movement of blacks. It was through the indoctrinations of Garvey that the Rastafarian movement was born (see Chapter 7).

Former U.S. Representative Shirley Chisholm was the first black woman to run for U.S. president and the first black woman in Congress; she is of West Indian descent, since her mother was from Barbados and her father from Guyana. The first black lieutenant governor of California, Mervyn Dymally, was from Trinidad, while Ronald Blackwood from Jamaica was the first black mayor in the state of New York (Mount Vernon). Basil Paterson, whose father was from Grenada and whose mother was from Jamaica, is a former secretary of state of New York. Civil rights activist Stokely Carmichael, originally from Trinidad, worked closely with Dr. Martin Luther King, Jr., during the 1960s. Roy Innis, a native of St. Croix, Virgin Islands, is currently the executive director of the Congress of Racial Equality. Una Clarke (newly elected a New York City councilwoman for the Flatbush section in Brooklyn) is originally from Jamaica. Colin Moore, a political activist and attorney, originally from Guyana, is presently one of the most controversial and highly valued attorneys among African people in New York State.

In entertainment, "the West Indian influence is reflected in the Afro-Caribbean and Reggae rhythms" (Whitaker, 1986, p. 140). Actor Harry Belafonte, whose mother was from Jamaica (where he lived for 5 years) and whose father was from Martinique, was and still is an activist. Sidney Poitier, an Academy Award-winning actor and director, was born in Florida but moved to Nassau, Bahamas, where he lived with his family until he was a teenager. The actress Cicely Tyson is of West Indian background, since her parents were immigrants from Nevis. Geoffrey Holder, originally from Trinidad, is a choreographer, actor, and director. Calvin Lockhart, a native of the Bahamas, moved to the United States at the age of 19 and shortly thereafter embarked on a modeling and acting career. Madge Sinclair, originally from Jamaica and the great-grandniece of Marcus Garvey, is a successful actress in both films and television. Grace Jones, originally from Jamaica, is both a singer and actress who migrated to the United States at age 12. Sheryl Lee Ralph, an actress, considers herself "Jamerican" because her mother is Jamaican, although her father is American. As a child, she spent much time on her mother's native island, and she attributes her success to her experiences in both cultures. Bob Marley of Jamaica "almost single handedly made Reggae into a household word around the globe" (Bernal, 1991, p. 4). Burke and Tompkins

(1991) say that "rap and hip hop music owes its beginning to Reggae music and that American rap artists were greatly influenced by local Reggae rappers" (p. 11). Some artists who fall under the reggae banner are Blondie, Eric Clapton, Heavy D, New Kids on the Block, and Queen Latifah. The Mighty Sparrow and the Lord Kitchener, "the fathers of Calypso," originally from Grenada and Trinidad, respectively, have contributed significantly to the entertainment industry worldwide, along with many other West Indian artists. One of the most fascinating musical instruments, the steel pan, was developed in Trinidad and is considered one of the wonders in the musical world.

In the arts and sciences, Sir Arthur Lewis, a Nobel Prize–winning economist and professor of political economics at Princeton University, is a native of St. Lucia. Derek Walcott, also from St. Lucia and also a Nobel Prize winner, has won worldwide acclaim as a great poet. American literature has been enriched through the writings of such West Indians such as Claude McKay, Jamaica Kincaid, Margaret Walker Alexander, and Arthur Schomberg (who also assembled one of the largest collections of African artifacts in the United States in the Schomberg Center for Research in Black Culture, a part of the New York Public Library). Etzer Chicoye, a native of Haiti, is a noted chemist and the director of research and development for the Miller Brewing Company in Milwaukee.

In the areas of sports and beauty are prominent figures such as Patrick Ewing, star center for the New York Knicks, originally from Jamaica; he moved to the United States at age 12 with his parents. In 1976, Hasley Crawford from Trinidad won the 100-meter race at the Olympics. The first black woman to win the Miss World title, Jennifer Hosten (1970), was from Grenada; the first black woman to win the Miss Universe title, Janelle Commissiong (1977), was from Trinidad.

Those are but a few West Indians who have contributed to the educational, political, social, and economic fabric of American society. Some West Indian immigrants have opened small businesses, and are sponsoring radio stations (such as WLIB and WBLS in New York City) and newspapers (such as the *Carib News*) so that West Indians can keep abreast of what is going on in their native countries. Still others are simply ensuring that their children make use of every opportunity, emphasizing education as the tool to liberation. Whatever they are doing, there is no doubt that these immigrants, by and large, are gaining the respect of other Americans for their determination and drive. There is every reason for these West Indian immigrants to share in the joy and pride that come from contributing significantly to many spheres of human endeavor.

POSSIBLE SOURCES OF CONFLICT BETWEEN AFRICAN AMERICANS AND AFRICAN WEST INDIAN AMERICANS

Some major differences between African Americans and African West Indian Americans were discussed at the beginning of this chapter. In addition, these two groups differ considerably in their perception of the possibility of upward social mobility. While both desire strongly to advance themselves, they differ in the extent to which they perceive themselves as having control over their destinies. In a society in which whites constitute the majority, African Americans believe that the rewards may never equal the effort. They contend that their skin color will always hinder upward mobility. Thus they tend to externalize failure, blaming a racist system. Many educated blacks never let their children forget the saying, "No matter what you achieve, you will always be a nigger." This attitude has resulted in a sort of a "learned helplessness" approach and a fear of putting forth too much in case one's efforts prove futile. On the other hand, African West Indian immigrants tend to internalize their failure. Thus they attribute their children's failure to a lack of effort. This attitude stems directly from having lived in a predominantly black society, where they see leaders who, through their own initiatives and efforts, have attained educational and sociopolitical upward mobility. Thus even uneducated West Indians from low socioeconomic backgrounds live with the hope and expectation that their children will do better than they did. West Indians believe that sacrifice and hard work can ultimately result in power, prominence, and affluence. They rarely endorse the idea that one's race will be a deterrent to political empowerment. Of course, the reality of American racism hits home when all efforts are made and one is still denied a position even though one is more qualified than one's white counterpart.

Another major conflict centers on the matter of ethnic definition. Americans have traditionally defined themselves as either black or white. Thus a light-skinned black person is seen as black here in the United States and experiences no discomfort in such a definition. However, the same individual residing in the West Indies may have been termed "West Indian white." Color distinctions in the West Indies range from dark-skinned African black at one end of the spectrum to light-skinned European white at the other, with many gradations in between. Thus phenotypically light-skinned persons who migrate from the West Indies and are suddenly told they are black, because American society does not recognize the existence of physically intermediate populations, find themseves in a dilemma. On their native islands, they might have had a higher status because of their "high-colored" complexion.

Further compounding this issue is the fact that until recently African Americans defined themselves by a color—black. West Indians, on the other hand, define themselves primarily by their nationality. In the West Indies, one is defined by a nationality (Jamaican, Trinidadian, etc.) or by a combination of race and nationality (e.g., a Negro from Trinidad or an East Indian from Guyana or a Chinese from Jamaica). Therefore, in the United States, black West Indian immigrants see themselves as West Indians first. This has angered black Americans, who have felt that the West Indians are refusing to identify with black Americans, and have accused them of being "clannish." Interestingly, in spite of their resentment and criticism of West Indians for defining themselves by nationality, many black Americans today prefer to define themselves culturally as African Americans. Thus there seems to be less conflict based on West Indians' maintaining their Caribbean cultural definition.

Of course, now there is the question of whether black West Indians should refer to themselves as African West Indian Americans or African Americans. Since West Indians have no intention of denying a major part of their history, the West Indian identification will prevail. It is my contention, however, that people of African ancestry will be much stronger as a people if they define themselves solely as Africans who simply are residing in America, in the West Indies, in Britain, in Canada, or in Africa. This will afford us a more global definition of ourselves and will allow us all to embrace all of our heritage.

A concern for black West Indian families is that in the American educational system, West Indian children are not considered immigrants (but are grouped with black American children), and are thus not offered extra educational services that other immigrants, such as Latino and Asian children, are given. This has led to the misclassification and misdiagnosis of West Indian children, resulting in the misplacement of such children in special education. Chapter 11 sheds further light on this matter.

Another source of conflict and misunderstanding between black Americans and West Indian immigrants is the question of citizenship. African Americans believe that if more black West Indians become citizens, this will increase the political opportunities for Africans as a whole. Many West Indians residing in the United States are not citizens. In some cases they are not eligible to become citizens because of their illegal status here; more recently, the Immigration Act of 1990 has opened the doors to European and Russian immigrants but limited the number of people from the less developed countries, such as the West Indies, who may enter. In other cases they are eligible, but simply refuse to do so. In the former instances, there is a process that one goes through to become a legal permanent resident. In the latter cases, Chapter 2 should help one to understand the dilemma that confronts all immigrants—the concept of biculturalism or living in two worlds. Relinquishing one's citizenship connotes, for some people, a denouncement of one's country. It is a very difficult decision, especially if a person is undecided about whether he or she plans to return home.

One individual who filled out the Immigrant Attitude Survey (Appendix 1V) summarized the dilemma of many West Indian immigrants:

> Firstly, growing up in the West Indies taught me that I was a Jamaican. Then upon entrance into the United States, I was immediately told I was a West Indian. While I was able to understand this concept geographically and intellectually, emotionally and historically I simply could not understand, because West Indian history did not give me an appreciation of the other West Indian islands. Then as soon as I got out in the wider society, I was told I am black and on top of that, American. Now, here am I dealing with my own grief of leaving my family behind, abandoning my culture, and someone is expecting me to assimilate all of this. I never knew what it was to be a black American, other than what the media in the West Indies taught me, which is the very same thing that was taught here in the United States. To me, a black American was a victim of racism, poor, underclass, and all of the other negatives that we all heard. Thus, for me to assume the role of a black American, meant the acceptance of those negative things about myself. No one wants to be associated with the negative. Now, through observation and self-education, I understand that there is so much more to being not only a black American, but an African. It took me about 10 years to understand it all. I immediately became a citizen of the United States, because I felt I wanted to be part of this process, this rich history. Today, I am so proud of my African culture and African people wherever we are.

The general feeling is that all immigrants must go through a process of adjustment before they feel comfortable becoming citizens of another country. African Americans view the reluctance of black West Indians to become citizens as a rejection of them. These feelings are understandable; for example, the West Indians are seen by African Americans as depriving them by taking their scholarships as minorities while refusing to strengthen their political power. But while this was a fairly accurate perspective as recently as five years ago, it is not the case now. Today more West Indians are becoming citizens and seeking political positions. It must be remembered that the West Indian immigrant is a relatively new migrant to the United States. Because most West Indian islands are either former British colonies or still part of the British Commonwealth, West Indians traditionally tended to migrate to Britain, where they were automatically considered citizens. The process of becoming a citizen must be taught to West Indians as part of their overall adjustment and therapy. As soon as a West Indian is eligible to become a citizen (which is at least five years after obtaining permanent residency), discussion about bcoming a citizen should be initiated. Chapter 12 on counseling can serve as a guide to address this matter.

The question about public assistance also needs to be addressed. It is said that black Americans utilize public assistance and black West Indians generally do not. Likewise, it is said that Puerto Ricans use public assistance and other Latino groups usually do not. One contributing factor here is that both black Americans and Puerto Ricans are U.S. citizens (Puerto Rico is a U.S. commonwealth), with all the attendant rights of citizenship. To obtain public assistance, one has to be a legal resident of the United States, but even permanent resident status does not entitle one to all forms of public assistance. In addition, all legal immigrants must document financial stability to show that they are not likely to become wards of the state for several years after entry. Finally, the very concept of public assistance is foreign to the average West Indian immigrant, whose native country does not have such a system.

Prior to entry into the United States, immigrants have to demonstrate that they are goal-focused and indicate how they will contribute to the social fabric of society. Thus Sowell's (1981) statement that West Indians "have been disproportionately overrepresented among Black professionals" (p. 564) is not surprising. Immigrants in general leave their native lands in order to do better; the ideal, of course, is to improve their educational and/or social standing. Thus added to the self-imposed pressure and pressure from friends and family back home is pressure from the U.S. government, which will not even permit residency if there is suspicion that an individual can become a parasite on the social system. Interestingly, this overrepresentation in the professions and willingness to work several jobs are not as prevalent in the West Indies themselves. An anecdote from some of the Nevisians to whom I administered the West Indian Attitude Survey (Appendix V) sheds further light on this matter. Many construction workers, originally from Trinidad, had been employed in

Nevis on a major building project. The Trinidadian workers were said to be "hard-working men who worked up until 10:00 every night," suggesting that the Trinidadians were more goal-focused and hard-working than the local Nevisians. I found this amusing, because had the very same workers been working in Trinidad, the likelihood of their putting in extra hours would have been slim. The behaviors displayed by the Nevisian workers were similar to those of the Trinidadian construction workers in Trinidad. The issue here was migration. Once the workers were in a foreign country, they recognized that nonchalant attitudes would be less acceptable in the host country. Thus voluntary migration in and of itself fosters a sense of direction, and a feeling of pride, motivation, and drive.

Along with this is the commonly raised issue that black West Indians will accept menial and low-paying jobs (such as domestic work) that black Americans would ordinarily reject, thereby making it more difficult for black Americans to lobby for better jobs and higher salaries. But it must be remembered that West Indian immigrants usually come from low socioeconomic backgrounds and often had much difficulty obtaining employment in their native lands. The West Indians see an opportunity to work not only one job, but two. Here are the means by which they can support not only the family members here in the United States, but also family members who were left behind in poverty.

On the other hand, history should shed light on the pain that black Americans experience at the thought of their wives or mothers being maids in someone else's home. It must be noted here that the concept of a maid in the West Indies is vastly different from the concept of a domestic in the United States. The average black middle-class family in the West Indies has helpers or maids in the home. A maid is seen more as a surrogate mother who disciplines the children, cares for the home, and even serves as a confidante for the woman whose husband is neglectful or abusive. Domestic service does not have the servile connotation in the West Indies that it has in the United States. Thus being employed as a domestic conjures up little or no historical pain for a West Indian woman, who sees it as serving two purposes—earning a living and obtaining permanent residency. Many domestics who do not have their permanent residency in the United States are sponsored by Americans and are able to obtain their green cards, their passports to legality.

Family roles constitute another area of conflict. In the United States, black women play a much stronger role in male–female relationships than they do in the West Indies. West Indian men are very strong figures who tend to have the final say in the way their families function. While their primary responsibility is to provide financially for their families, the women's primary responsibility is one of childrearing and home care. These roles are clearly defined, and everyone understands his or her position. Needless to say, migration to the United States, where black men are depicted as less dominant in the family, disrupts the status quo. Marital and familial conflict may erupt when these traditional sex roles are reversed. At times the woman may have to be the breadwinner, because obtaining employment tends to be easier for the migrant woman than the migrant man. The man may be expected to stay at home and care for the family. This role shift may not be a problem if the woman nonetheless continues to accept the traditional perspective of family life. Chapter 12 explores some of these conflicts and possible therapeutic resolutions. However, in light of this rigid family role definition, black West Indian men are angry at black American men for their "passivity" (clearly a myth), and black West Indian women are fascinated at the independence of black American women. These issues play themselves out in many situations, leading at times to bonding or conflict.

Another issue of concern for African Americans is the perception that white Americans give "preferential treatment" to African West Indians because they see the West Indians as "not hung up as much on race." Because the racism historically experienced by black Americans was not experienced in the same intensity by West Indians, the West Indians' tolerance or ignorance of institutionalized racism is understandable. However, once individuals have been in this country long enough to be aware of the history of the U.S. race relations, they are able to identify with the African Americans' experiences.

One can appreciate, after viewing these differences, that the therapeutic approaches to working with African Americans and African West Indian immigrants must be different. The "healthy cultural paranoia" and "suspicion" (Boyd-Franklin, 1989) that are seen in black American clients are not, for the most part, present in black West Indians. Thus, while West Indians' failure to talk may have to do with embarrassment, for African Americans, it may be largely due to "a direct learned survival response that Blacks are socialized to adapt from an early age" (Boyd-Franklin, 1989, p. 19).

To sum up, although black West Indians share the African legacy and the historical experiences of slavery with African Americans, and although the two groups possess some cultural similarities, there are many differences that have an impact on West Indians' adjustment. A therapist who is remiss in addressing these differences may hinder the process of acculturation for West Indian immigrants. In contrast, highlighting some of the differences may help African Americans and black West Indian immigrants to engage in honest and meaningful dialogue, as they continue to get to know each other and to discover fundamental similarities. While the focus should always be on their common destiny as Africans, reclaiming pride in their group histories, enhancing appreciation for group differences, and preserving individual uniqueness must also be recognized and encouraged.

CHAPTER 9

West Indian Families in Britain

In December 1990 I contacted the Department of Education and Science in Great Britain, requesting assistance in conducting a research study on West Indian immigrant families. The department directed me to the local educational authorities for school provision in many parts of England where there are large numbers of West Indian immigrants. Interestingly, in response to my letter, the inspectorate's office informed me that "the word 'immigrant' is hardly relevant to the vast majority of pupils whose families originated in the West Indies." They went on to explain that because their parents were born in Britain and they were themselves born in Britain, they do not consider themselves immigrants. It was suggested that another term be used. In my personal interviews with the participants in the study, I referred to them as "British," "black British," "English," or "black English," refraining from using the word "immigrant." While the inspectorate was correct in stating that the word "immigrant" was inappropriate, for the most part West Indians residing in Britain do not consider themselves Englishmen or Englishwomen, black Englishmen or black Englishwomen, black British, or simply British. As Hinds (1966) put it, "people lose respect for us when we let them think that we want to be Black Englishmen" (quoted in Scobie, 1972, p. 296). West Indians define themselves as "Afro-Caribbean" or simply "black," even if they are the second generation to be born in Britain. Mabey (1986) referred to children of West Indian heritage as "black Afro-Caribbean." One gentleman helped elucidate this matter when he told me that while everyone in the United States is in fact an immigrant except the Native Americans, everyone in Britain is British except the immigrants, who are of West Indian, Asian, or African heritage. The insularity of the British and British institutional racism have rendered West Indians "foreigners" in spite of their contributions to the United Kingdom.

The West Indian movement to Britain began during World War II, when the country needed additions to its labor force. News spread back to the islands that a better life could be had in the "mother country," since in the West Indies there was a "shortage of employment and limited opportunity for advancement via the educational system" (Lamur & Speckmann, 1975, p. 34). Thus in the early 1950s a stream of migrants went to Britain. It is also thought that the McCarran–Walter Act of 1952, which blocked West Indian immigration into the United States, was partly responsible for this increased West Indian migration to the United Kingdom. It is estimated that 20,000 to 33,000 immigrants a year entered the United Kingdom between 1950 and 1955.

From about 1955 to 1959, "British citizens reacted strongly to this Black invasion and their government moved to halt the movement by hasty legislation" (Marshall, 1982, p. 9). The Commonwealth Immigration Act of 1962 controlled immigration to the United Kingdom. However, 168,000 West Indians entered the United Kingdom between 1960 and 1962 before the British closed their doors. In 1965, the White Paper on Immigration from the Commonwealth established the principle that "Black people were in themselves a problem and that [the] fewer of them in the UK, the better it would be" (Marshall, 1982, p. 9). The Nationality Bill further crystallized the sentiments of the British government toward West Indians, removing any doubts about their status: They were "aliens, Black colonial subjects who are not wanted in the Mother Country" (Marshall, 1982, p. 10). Furthermore, during the Thatcher administration, a proposal was made to help West Indians return to their native countries. Since West Indian migrants had sold all their material goods and left their jobs before migrating to the United Kingdom, repatriation was not economically, politically, or morally feasible.

Moreover, in 1987 all West Indians, regardless of how long they had been residing in the United Kingdom, had to register themselves as citizens. West Indians, who had thought of themselves as citizens already (because of the dependent relationship that their countries of origin had to the British crown, prior to their migration to the United Kingdom), were insulted by this. Many of them refused to come forward, since they had resided in Britain for most of their lives. Furthermore, the government decided that even persons born in

Britain would not automatically be considered citizens unless both their parents were citizens or their parents' country of origin still had affinity to the British crown. Individuals whose parents are from countries that have gained their independence, such as Jamaica, Trinidad and Tobago, Barbados, Guyana, Grenada, St. Vincent and the Grenadines, Antigua and Barbuda, St. Lucia, and St. Kitts and Nevis, are not considered citizens even if they are born in the United Kingdom. "Such a child could be defined as a West Indian immigrant" (Mabey, 1981, p. 84), and his or her passport would read "right to abode." For such individuals to become citizens, they have to apply to the Home Office, where their applications will be considered like all others. The cost for naturalization on the grounds of residence is approximately 255 pounds; naturalization on the grounds of marriage costs about 225 pounds. West Indians very much resent what they see as unnecessary expenses, and feel they should be granted citizenship by being born in Britain. Granting citizenship is strictly up to the Home Office. There is also no set legal standard (as in the United States) that one is guaranteed citizenship because one's spouse is a citizen.

The anger that West Indians feel toward the British is quite understandable, since the United States, Canada, France, and the Netherlands (other major host or "mother" countries to West Indian immigrants) grant citizenship to all individuals born in the country. These laws and attitudes shed light on why West Indians do not feel that they have equality in Britain, as was to be expected, according to the Hunt Committee's report (Hunt, 1967). This report stated that the second and subsequent generations of "colored British" would naturally be expected to be treated equally and to have the same opportunity as other British citizens.

THE BRITISH EDUCATION SYSTEM AND WEST INDIANS

Mabey (1986) found that many of the West Indian students she studied in London were still not achieving the basic five O levels (equivalent to a high school diploma) that are required for many jobs and are needed for higher education or training. School officials still direct West Indian students to programs for the less intelligent; therefore, few West Indian students go on to university. Most are relegated to low-paying, menial jobs, and many work in factories or in offices as clerks. In addition, the educational system is geared toward the academically oriented, and those pursuing elite professions can really benefit, but there are few vocational schools that teach trades.

Students who do not obtain a high school diploma usually have little opportunity for upward mobility. This is very different from the United States, where nonacademic students can learn viable trades that yield high salaries.

Giles (1977), in examining the West Indian experience in British schools, found that teachers' stereotypes and expectations about West Indian children influenced the way they interacted with them. According to Giles, teacher interviews revealed a number of negative stereotypes, such as that West Indian children lose their tempers faster and explode more quickly. One teacher in Giles's study said she had observed that West Indian children became extremely excitable in large groups, and therefore kept them in smaller groups where they were more manageable. She attributed their behavior to the culture at home. The teachers in Giles's study even had more negative attitudes and feelings toward West Indian students than toward white disadvantaged students. This state of affairs is unfortunate, because when West Indian immigrants first migrated they had great hope for the future of their children, because they had confidence in the rectitude of the "motherland." The West Indian parents who participated in Giles's study said they had hoped that their children would get a university degree, since this would have been difficult to do in their homelands.

Many reasons can be offered as to why West Indian children even today experience failure in the school system, including the "hidden curriculum," the influence of environmental factors, teacher expectations, and the lack of parent advocacy. Young and Bagley (1979) found that the majority of the West Indian children in their study were seen negatively by their teachers. When children are not viewed favorably by teachers, and when they are not encouraged to pursue their professional dreams, they will not be stimulated to their maximum potential. Research has shown that when teachers expect that certain children will show greater intellectual development, those children do; when teachers' expectations are low, a self-fulfilling prophecy may take effect, and even children with high ability may not succeed (Rosenthal & Jacobson, 1968). Eighty-two percent of the adolescent and young adult West Indians who participated in my study described the British school system as "discouraging." They claimed they were "ignored, ridiculed, and belittled"; that they were not given the proper career guidance; and that they were not put in the necessary courses for pursuing a university education. They also claimed that they did not feel part of the British educational system, since a multicultural curriculum has not been implemented to defeat the "hidden curriculum" that operates in most schools. This curriculum teaches all children that the black student comes from a culture where there is no positive literature, and that the system is dominated by literature and history from a white perspective. The participants felt that in spite of the contributions of West Indians to history, art, technology, philosophy, and science, students are still not exposed to the work of Africans, Caribbeans, Afro-Americans, and black British writers. In like manner, the participants felt that while blatant racist images may not be as prevalent today as they were 20 years ago, excluding blacks from the curriculum is equally racist.

Teachers, especially black teachers, need to advocate for a multicultural and antiracist curriculum, since this is one of the tools that can defeat the hidden curriculum. Teaching about the rich culture and history of the West Indian heritage can enhance the positive self-esteem of West Indian students. Continuing to treat African and Caribbean literature as an anomaly, instead of integrating it into the main curriculum in all subject areas, is dangerously narrow-minded. Without any cultural anchorage, and with the perpetuation of a distorted historical reality, West Indian students may be on a route to self-negation.

Furthermore, although West Indian children speak with a British accent and speak English at school, most of their grandparents—and to some extent even their parents—still speak Creole. "Our parents never let us forget our historical dialect and culture," said one adolescent. However, in Britain, the Creole language has been viewed as the language of "backward" people. Several of the participants painfully recalled being told to "speak English," resulting in their being embarrassed by their West Indian dialect. Gibson (1986), describing his interviews with young West Indians, explains how frustrated many children became because they were put down directly and indirectly by their teachers. The teacher who is given no training in analyzing Creole language features (see Chapter 11) simply views Creole as "baby talk." As a result, many West Indian children as recently as five years ago were still being placed in classes for the educationally subnormal, because many of the tests were language-based. The implication is that standard English is normal and the Creole language is subnormal and deficient, rather than different (see Chapters 11 and 15). Since "West Indian parents express a very high regard for education and are keen to aid their children's schooling" (Yekwai, 1988, p. 19), it is amazing that many West Indian children were and still are seen as educational failures. Interestingly, the Plowden report (Plowden, 1967)—a report, in response to an outcry, that revealed an overall underachievement among children of working-class background in the British school system—placed the blame for their failure on them and their families (Yekwai, 1988).

In any event, teacher expectation and the biased curriculum are not the only explanations of black children's underachievement in the British schools. Studies have shown that in spite of the democratization of education in Britain over the last 40 years, social class inequalities have persistently affected educational performance (Saakana & Pearse, 1986). In addition, other environmental factors, such as poor housing, may affect educational performance. Though poverty is neither desirable nor ennobling, it ought not to produce serious deficiency in one's cognitive development. The material environment, however, helps to shape aspirations, self-esteem, ambition, and life goals.

THE WEST INDIAN FAMILY IN BRITAIN

A factor that cannot be overlooked in examining the underachievement of black children of West Indian heritage is the changing role of the West Indian family. While in the West Indies the extended family is the norm, in Britain, as in the United States, the nuclear family is the norm. In the West Indies, aunts, uncles, grandparents, godparents, and friends all play an important role in childrearing (see Chapter 3). In Britain, "relatives and friends are seen as comparatively separate and uninfluential" (Gibson, 1985, p. 46). Given the family dynamics in the West Indian culture, it is vitally important to work with the whole family in treatment and not with the children alone, even if the children may have been identified initially as the reason for referral.

A source of major familial conflict among West Indians in Britain is the issue of discipline. British children are given more liberty, and West Indian parents are expected to give up disciplining children in their traditional way (see Chapter 12). This presents a tremendous problem for parents and grandparents, who have to adjust to concepts such as child abuse and neglect. Giles (1977) found that teachers described West Indian parents as "more autocratic." Gibson's (1986) testimonials from young West Indians showed that some children felt that it was difficult to talk to their parents, who did not understand the system and blamed them for "not trying hard enough."

Many parents fear the police will harass their children who socialize on the street in the summer. Police, in their attempts to combat street crime, tend to arrest those they perceive as loiterers; since it is customary in West Indian culture to use the street as a congregating point, West Indian adolescents are victimized. Parents expect their children to stay indoors to avoid police harassment, and the children rebel against their parents' fear. This results in major parent–child conflict in the home. Mental health workers' condemnation of the parents and alignment with the children certainly compound the parents' fear of the social/legal sytem, which they perceive as being against them. Teaching parents alternative ways to discipline and communicate more effectively with their children ought to be a focus in treatment (see Chapter 15).

Women are frequently the heads of the households, because it is more difficult for men to obtain employment. Raspberry (1991) commented on the findings of Pryde, a Washington economic consultant who attended a conference on black economic empowerment in England in the spring of 1991. In summarizing Pryde's findings, Raspberry (1991) noted "that the barriers to job opportunities for Black men are very obviously discriminatory policies, that well trained Blacks in England today cannot find work and have to turn to lesser jobs" (p. 35). It may affect a male's sense of self to be made to feel inferior in his own home. In England, stereotypes such as "lazy" and "absent from the home" are applied to black men, particularly black men of West Indian heritage. To blame the victim and overlook the reality that the black male has little access to the job market is to be naive with respect to institutionalized racism. Boyd-Franklin (1989) attributes much of this "subtle form of discrimination" to the fears about black men. These negative stereotypes (erroneous as they may be) have a debilitating effect on black males and their ability to function as husbands, fathers, and workers.

Many have argued that this sort of stereotyping seems to be more of a class factor than a racial one. In other words, middle-class black fathers are more involved in childrearing and in decision making than fathers from the lower socioeconomic levels. A very important point to note in working with British families of West Indian heritage is that there is a small percentage of upwardly mobile West Indians who are middle-class and want to be recognized for their achievement. What affects the West Indian educated middle class most is the fact that even to this day, little distinction is made between black people of different classes and different educational levels. The race and class systems in England are very rigid. To endorse the "class, not race" myth in English society is to be naive about the insidious nature of racism. It is very difficult for blacks to be accepted among the upper and middle classes. And even when they are, the question still looms as to whether a black person can feel psychologically and socially secure in his or her ability to maintain those socioeconomic gains in a racist society such as Britain. As one woman I interviewed said, "You have to prove yourself even if you are educated and have acquired wealth. You have to prove that you are worthy of the upper and middle classes."

The British system is very elitist, and elite is associated with white. This attitude is embedded deeply in the psyche of the people. There is no affirmative action or quota system in Britain. Although there are laws in place in the United Kingdom to combat racism (such as the Race Relations Act of 1976), there is still a need for the clear application of the law and for a clear judicial commitment to racial equality. One participant in my study said, "If we really had legal systems in place which were taken seriously, we might have been more powerful as a group." This statement to a large extent helps in understanding the insidiousness of racism in Britain. The British have had fewer encounters with people of African heritage residing in their country as citizens than Americans have had. The Africans who were brought to the United States as slaves remained there and have since contributed to the American society. For the most part, blacks came to Britain only during and after World War II, and today make up only 5% of the population of the United Kingdom. Britain never really felt that it had to accommodate blacks, since it saw them as temporary laborers who might one day return to their native lands. Thus there was never any strong lobbying force to challenge the status quo. Raspberry (1991) noted that that the black British "are about a generation behind their U.S. counterparts in terms of creating the public and political awareness necessary for change" (p. 35).

In Britain, West Indians and other blacks have experienced political, economic, social, and educational inequalities and, given their numbers, have been unable to effect change. The media are certainly not as flamboyant and do not strive for sensationalism as much as in the United States. However, to some extent such sensationalism is needed to bring attention to the racism. But in spite of the institutionalized racism that exists in the United Kingdom, blacks do not have a sense of complete helplessness. The strength of blacks in the United Kingdom is evident in their unyielding fight for equality and their tireless effort in questioning and demanding a fair education and a fair social/legal system for all people.

Unfortunately, in spite of these efforts, many parents are still unaware of the agencies that can serve as advocates for them. They need to familiarize themselves with the various schools and their entry requirements. Parents also need to find out about the benefits, scholarships, and medical care that are available in their communities, as well as to set up social and recreational activities for their children in their communities. The most important gain for parents would come from their involvement in the education system. Attending parent–

teacher meetings, getting involved in curriculum development and parent associations or parent support groups, and monitoring homework are all necessary. If parents are unable to assist their children themselves, they should explore the possibility of hiring a tutor.

MENTAL HEALTH/RELIGION AND WEST INDIANS

Because a person's medical records remain on file for 40 years in Britain, many people, particularly those of African heritage, are very suspicious of mental health workers. In general, West Indians view psychologists and other mental health workers in an adverse way. One politician who was a participant in my study said, "Historically, blacks who opposed the system were institutionalized, because militancy can easily be viewed as aggression and mental derangement." Therefore, West Indians very rarely use mental health services unless they are forced to because of problems with their children. The extended family, the churches, and self-healing are preferred alternatives for the person of West Indian background. Many still believe that evil spirits are the causes of mental illness, and ministers in the churches are used to rid one of the evil. Generally, West Indians in Britain do not use spiritual healers and exorcists as much as they do in the West Indies or even in the United States, because it is difficult for them to practice there. Many black West Indians have moved away from Catholicism and have joined the Church of God. This affords them a more sociopolitical expression of their culture and music, with the church becoming more than a spiritual experience. Thus, unlike the churches in the West Indies (which are separate from politics), but like black churches in the United States, the black churches in the United Kingdom are used as bases for rising politicians. So in the West Indian communities of the United Kingdom, religion plays a significant role in the social and political life of the people.

INTERGROUP DIFFERENCES

People of color in the United Kingdom are not a monolithic group, despite the fact that Britain usually lumps them all together as "black" (see Chapter 5). There are cultural differences among black people of West Indian heritage, black people originally from Africa, and people of East Indian heritage. Unlike the East Indians, who are seen as businesspeople because over time they have acquired a certain amount of business acumen, West Indians are viewed more in a social sense. Thus West Indian music is quite influential, especially reggae and to a lesser extent calypso. Africans are more known for their culture—for instance, their artistry. Even today, much conflict exists among all groups. The West Indians believe that the Africans view them as "slave babies" (because black West Indians, like African Americans, were sold into slavery). Both the Africans and the West Indians believe that the Asians do not think of themselves as "black" unless they fall victim to racism; at such times, it is thought, they claim racism and are able to solicit the support of black groups. Unfortunately, there is much intergroup hostility, anger, and frustration; West Indians believe that these are fostered by governmental policies, which thrive on the divide-and-conquer concept. It is thought that East Indians are given more opportunities to open their own businesses, and this creates resentment in other immigrant communities. Intergroup harmony must be fostered if a true coalition and a strong lobbying force are to be formed.

Although interisland differences existed when West Indians first migrated to the United Kingdom, for the most part this is not the case now. Most islanders (regardless of their country of origin) bond together. However, Jamaicans do have a distinctly different style that gives them the status of "Jamaicans," as opposed to the other islanders, who are seen simply as "West Indians." In general, it is racism that helps West Indians to preserve their cultural identity in spite of having been in Britain for as much as half a century.

CHAPTER 10

West Indian Families in Canada

The history of West Indian migration to Canada began with the slaves who were imported into New France and Nova Scotia in 1796. In 1795, the Maroon slaves in Jamaica (who continued to be in constant conflict with the British government; see Chapter 6) surrendered their arms after a war had erupted with the British, and were exiled to Nova Scotia. The Maroons were offered employment on the outskirts of Halifax, but their continued appeals to London to leave Halifax later resulted in their remigration to Sierra Leone, West Africa, in 1800 (Walker, 1984).

Over the next century the migration to Canada from the West Indies was limited to a few dozen families who went to Victoria, a few to Nova Scotia, and some to Ontario. Only at the end of the nineteenth century did the number of West Indian migrants begin to increase, because there was a need for workers in the coal mines in Sydney, Nova Scotia. During World War I several hundred more West Indians were recruited as laborers, primarily for the Cape Breton mines (Walker, 1984). After the war, when the veterans returned and resumed their jobs, the West Indians moved to Toronto and Montreal in search of employment. They were later joined by their families and other West Indians. By 1921 there were approximately 1,200 West Indians residing in Toronto and 400 in Montreal (Walker, 1984). Migration ceased after the early 1920s because of the global racism of the early twentieth century. Blacks were described as "lazy, sexually over-active, criminally inclined and genetically inferior" (Walker, 1984, p. 9). After World War II Britain had a demand for unskilled workers, so more than 300,000 West Indians migrated there to escape poverty in the West Indies. Thousands also went to the United States until a restricted annual quota was imposed by the McCarran–Walter Act of 1952.

After America closed its doors in the mid-1950s, West Indians attempted to enter Canada. However, Canada did not relax the racial bias in its immigration policy against blacks and Chinese. Concerned about the increased interest in their country, Canadian authorities tightened their policy to curb the flow of nonwhite immigrants. In 1955 an experimental migration policy, known as the West Indian Domestic Scheme, brought 100 domestics from the West Indies to work in Canadian homes. To be eligible for this program, an individual had to pass a medical examination, be a single female between the ages of 18 and 35, and have at least an eighth-grade education. Applicants were interviewed by a team of Canadian immigration officials who visited the islands once per year specifically to recruit domestic workers. A significant feature of West Indian immigration to Canada in comparison to the other regions of the world has been the above-average proportion of women who migrate alone. In Canada in 1981, the ratio of males per 100 females was 83 (Dumas, 1989).

Upon their arrival in Canada, the women were granted landed-immigrant status (equivalent to a green card) and were expected to work in a home for about one year. After a year's service, they had the option of finding work in another field or remaining in domestic labor. A major problem that resulted from this scheme was that many of the applicants were not really domestics in their native countries, but were instead teachers, nurses, secretaries, and so forth who used this scheme as a way to gain legitimate status in Canada. Thus many of them opted to leave domestic service after one year, and the shortage of domestic workers continued. The government, in turn, stopped automatically granting landed-immigrant status to domestics, instead issuing temporary employment visas. This program was different in that each visa was issued for a particular kind of job, for a specific employer, and for a definite period of time. If any circumstances changed, the holder of the visa had to report immediately to the Employment and Immigration Commission or run the risk of being deported (Silvera, 1986).

By 1962, there was considerable pressure to reform the immigration policies. Newly independent West Indian countries were critical of the racial restrictions, and in 1962 revised Canadian immigration regulations were issued. The racially discriminatory provisions of the Immigration Act of Canada were lifted, and potential immigrants were allowed or denied entry on the basis of a point system that measured skills, training, and education. Therefore, with the exception of the entrants under the Domestic Scheme, priority was given to West Indian immigrants who were professionals or skilled workers. Most of the West Indian immigrants currently in Canada (75%) entered after 1962.

In general, migration from the West Indies to Canada has been relatively small in comparison to migration to Britain and the United States. Only 188,000 people entered between 1946 and 1979 (Henry, 1982). However, since the Canadian census asks only for the last country of residence, West Indians who have come to Canada via Britain are counted as British. In addition, West Indians of Asian origin are classified at times as Asian rather than West Indian. Toronto and its surrounding areas have the largest numbers of West Indians, many of whom came under the Domestic Scheme. Quebec, because of its Francophone policy, has attracted migrants from the French-speaking countries, such as Haiti and the French West Indies. Ontario has immigrants from all over, with West Indians comprising a substantial number.

Because of the size of the country, Jamaicans have predominated in the movements to Britain, United States, and Canada. About two-fifths of the West Indian population in Canada is of Jamaican origin. To a large extent, much to the chagrin of the other islanders, "Jamaican" has become the generic term for "West Indians" in Canada. However, Trinidad and Guyana are significant contributors as well. This may be attributable to the contribution that the Canadian Presbyterian Mission made in educating East Indian children in Trinidad and Guyana when their parents refused to send them to public school for fear they would be converted to Christianity (see Chapter 5). Thus the relationship between the Mission and the East Indians from these countries has been a long and positive one. Barbadian migration to Canada was a pilot scheme in response to the need for female farm workers. In general, migration to Canada from the West Indies has taken place for economic reasons. The usual pattern has been to leave the dependent children behind until the parent (sponsor) can get established, with a place to live and some economic security.

WEST INDIANS IN THE EDUCATION SYSTEM

West Indian children in the Canadian school system experience discrimination primarily because of cultural differences between the home and school environments, teaching styles, and language factors (Valere-Meredith, 1989). Even though many of the children of West Indian backgrounds speak with a Canadian accent, "the language spoken by the vast majority is called Creole by linguists and patois by West Indians" (Valere-Meredith, 1989, p. 2). Since not all islands have the same dialect, it is difficult for teachers to comprehend some of the newly arrived West Indian immigrant children. Chapter 11 sheds some light on misclassification resulting from language differences, and Chapter 15 examines techniques that teachers and speech pathologists can use to more accurately assess West Indian students' dialectical differences.

In general, beyond issues of language, West Indian children are accustomed to more structure and to strict discipline. Thus when children wait for guidance and interpretation from the teacher, teachers perceive this as a delaying tactic, resulting at times in the children being retained in a grade or receiving negative reports. The problem is compounded because West Indian parents' cultural upbringing has taught them to respect teachers and the school system at large. They tend to blame the children for their alleged failings and very rarely confront teachers about evaluations. As far as West Indian parents are concerned, once they have made an initial visit to the school to enroll their child, it is then up to him or her to maximize the use of the immense opportunities (Anderson & Grant, 1987).

Solomon (1992) discusses the effect of the Canadian education system and its contribution to separatism. He emphasizes that in the Canadian tracking system, whereby children are sorted, classified, and grouped according to their abilities, aptitudes, and needs, students from racial minority groups and low socioeconomic status are more likely than others to be in the lowest academic tracks. Of course, the result of being in the lowest track is that these children's career aspirations are limited because the work force prefers higher track, dominant group workers (Solomon, 1992).

WEST INDIAN FAMILY ROLES

Whereas in the West Indies family roles follow rigid lines of demarcation, with women assuming the childrearing roles (see Chapter 3), there is a blurring of marital roles in Canada. Parent–child role diffusion, child discipline, single parenting, and the absence of the extended family as a result of migration also create changes in family roles. In spite of the drive for skilled workers and professionals, immigration restrictions and the fact that available jobs tend to be in female-dominated areas have still made it easier for women to migrate first (see Chapter 2). This meant that between 1962 and 1970 women outnumbered men from the West Indian regions. Unfortunately, it took the women many years to save enough money to bring their families to Canada. As a result, the children viewed their extended families, in particular their grandparents, as their parents. This created much difficulty in establishing healthy parent–child relationships upon the arrival of the children in Canada. In addition, the children often had to adjust to new siblings and/or a new stepfather.

To compound the problem further, in the case of the husband who migrates after his wife, there is the issue of household chores. Traditionally, West Indian women do all or most of the housework. A woman who works full-time outside the home and is still expected to take full responsibility for housework tends to resent this double responsibility and to become frustrated and angry, further exacerbating the already stressful experience of migration. In the past 10 years, Canada has seen an increase in the migration of nuclear families, which mitigates some of the problems with the changes in familial roles. However, the support of the extended family, which is counted on in the West Indies, remains nonexistent. Chapter 12 addresses these issues in greater detail.

A positive aspect of family life is the high value West Indian parents place on achievement. "Even in the poorest of families, parents have high aspirations for their children and each generation encourages the next to move a step ahead" (Christiansen, Thornley-Brown, & Robinson, 1984, p. 47). In their study of West Indians in Toronto, Christiansen and associates found that while 52% of the parents in the sample were unskilled workers, over 80% of their children aspired to skilled, clerical, or professional jobs.

EMPLOYMENT PATTERN

Most West Indians are employed as unskilled or clerical workers, closely followed by those in the health fields (such as nurses) and then by those in entrepreneurial, managerial, and administrative jobs. In general, it has been reported that West Indians in comparison to other ethnic groups still have "low status jobs, earn lower incomes and experience more job insecurity even when education and skills are controlled" (Henry, 1982, p. 38). West Indians were found to have more education and skill than Portuguese and Italians, but they still earn less money and experience more job insecurity. Even for the men who are in high-status jobs in the medical and health fields, "it does not appear to alter their overall income significantly" (Henry, 1982, p. 39).

Racial discrimination is a major contributing factor to this economic inequality. Subtle as these forms of discrimination may seem (for instance, word-of-mouth advertising), they have created barriers to members of racial and ethnic minorities. The use of such screening devices as requesting "Canadian experience" for jobs that require more knowledge than "Canadian experience" itself, and the principle of "last hired, first fired," are a few of the employment practices that affect ethnic minorities more than most other groups. One individual who responded to the Immigrant Attitude Survey (Appendix IV) highlighted the difficulty in attaining pay commensurate with his qualifications: "I was shocked when I graduated from university and realized that my white friends who did not go on to university were more successful financially and had less difficulty obtaining jobs than I did." Of note is the below-average number of West Indians who are self-employed and employing others. Even Caribbean immigrants who immigrated to Canada between 1960 and 1969, and therefore had time to establish themselves, were much less likely to be employers or to be self-employed than were corresponding immigrants from elsewhere (4.2% compared with 7.7%) (Dumas, 1989).

RACISM AND WEST INDIANS

Whereas in the West Indies West Indians of color are in the majority, in Canada they are in the minority. Although people of color comprise less than 5% of the population, racist sentiment against nonwhites nonetheless exists and has been a major problem in cities such as Toronto and Montreal, manifested in beatings, harassment, the destruction of South Asian places of worship, police brutality, distribution of hate literature, and physical and verbal fights in schools between whites and nonwhites. The view of West Indians as "lazy, slow-moving, and uneducated" is not consistent with the educated and hard-working skilled workers many have proven to be. This racism can be very traumatic, since West Indians in their native lands were not exposed to the same level of racism so commonly experienced in Britain, the United States, and Canada. Often they feel powerless, react with denial, and become vulnerable to stress and crisis. In his study, however, James (1990) found that youths felt that racism can be overcome by "developing the right attitude—that nothing will stop them from succeeding" (p. 76).

In response to this direct racism, a variety of task forces and committees have been formed by governmental, institutional, religious, and private organizations. There is even a special "ethnic squad" on the police force and race relations groups in the schools to recommend sanctions against teachers and students who are guilty of racist behaviors. Even the media have been forced to examine their racist imagery and to combat racism through educational training, symposia, and so forth.

INTERGROUP DIFFERENCES

In addition to the pressures imposed externally, there are social problems among the various nonwhite groups. First, there is tension between those of African and those of East Indian descent, as described in earlier chapters. Moreover, there is a significant amount of fragmentation among blacks themselves, because black West Indians tend to disassociate themselves from Canadian blacks. Chapter 8 explores cultural differences between African Americans and black West Indian Americans, and reviewing this chapter can shed some light on the Canadian black–West Indian black tensions. West Indian Canadians feel that they are superior to Canadian blacks, whom they view as nonachieving and unambitious. Canadian blacks view West Indians as haughty and arrogant, and feel insulted when they are asked, "And what island are you from?"

In Montreal and elsewhere in Quebec, there is also segmentation among the Canadian blacks, the black French-speaking migrants (such as the Haitians), and the black migrants from the English-speaking West Indies. The Haitians are not accepted the way French speakers of European origin are, because their color sets them apart from this group. Thus there is tension between the Haitians and Quebecois. Another problem is that the Haitians have not aggressively supported the French Canadians against the English Canadians, because they define themselves as Haitians first. Anglophone West Indians also remain aloof from the French Canadian struggle. The relationship between Anglophone and Francophone West Indians is hindered by the language barrier; although some of the English-speaking West Indians assisted in the fight against the deportation of illegal Haitian immigrants, there are few social relations between the two language groups. Then, of course, there are the island nationalisms, manifested in such groups as the Jamaican and the Trinidadian associations. Moreover, there is the dichotomy between those who define themselves primarily by their color and those who define themselves primarily by their parents' culture of origin.

All these factors—the segmentation of the West Indians as a whole, racism, the stressors of migration itself—contribute to the fact that West Indians remain on the periphery as marginal members in a society dominated by whites. In spite of their high motivational levels, and despite their achievement and upward mobility and their coming together annually for Toronto's Caribbean carnival (Caribana), total integration into the mainstream of Canadian society is difficult for West Indians, who are not treated as first-class citizens even if they were born there. There is still a sense of a lack of connectedness to a broader Canadian society. Perhaps to expect the merging of so many groups, races, and nationalities in any one society is unrealistic. Perhaps if immigrants could attain a harmonious climate, where there is equal access to employment and to social and educational opportunities, regardless of racial or ethnic affiliations, they would be content to live with their differences.

ASSESSMENT ISSUES, MAJOR TREATMENT THEORIES, AND A MODEL FOR INTERVENTION

CHAPTER 11

Assessment: Educational, Linguistic, Psychological

Because of the new influx of West Indian immigrants, it is vitally important that psychologists and educators begin to examine cultural differences in evaluating children from the West Indies. This chapter explores techniques in assessing West Indians educationally, linguistically, and psychologically.

EDUCATIONAL ASSESSMENT

In assessing the educational functioning of the recently arrived West Indian immigrant child, one must be aware not only of different pronunciation but also of different spellings of certain words. Because most of the English-speaking West Indies were once British colonies, characteristically British spelling is used, such as "-our" instead of "-or" (e.g., "honour") and "-re" instead of "-er" (e.g., "centre"). West Indians no longer use the British "-ise" but have adopted the American "-ize" (e.g., "organize"). The word "program" in the West Indies is still spelled the British way, "programme." The West Indian immigrant child has to learn that words are spelled differently in the United States, a process that takes approximately three years and requires excellent short- and long-term visual and auditory memory.

In recording date of birth, one must be aware that in the West Indies, as in Britain, the day is listed first, then the month, then the year. So a birth date of July 16, 1980, is recorded as 16/7/80. Based on this cultural difference, many American examiners have stated that West Indian children do not know their birth dates and confuse the months with the days. Some educators have recorded incorrect birth dates in children's records; for example, 10/6 means October 6 according to the American convention, but June 10 according to the British.

Part 2 of the WICAB (Appendix II) describes in detail the process of placing West Indian children by grade.

LINGUISTIC ASSESSMENT

What makes West Indian immigrants particularly difficult to assess is their language. Many educators and clinicians question whether these children speak English. Although the official language in the West Indies is English because of the former colonial relationship with Britain, West Indians speak a variety of dialects, such as West Indian Creole or Haitian Creole, which are basically combinations of English, Spanish, French, and African languages. They are a sort of "broken" English, quite different from the British or American speech. In their native countries West Indians are taught to read and write standard English, but they speak West Indian Creole in the classroom. Thus the children's dialect, pronunciation, and accent are different. The fact that some words are pronounced differently means that on an oral spelling test some children may have difficulty spelling words that they know but did not recognize because of the different pronunciation. For example, for the West Indian child, the "er" in the word "sister" is pronounced as an "a"—thus "sista"; the "h" in "th" may be unvoiced—so "three" may be pronounced "tree"; "sk" may be said as "x" or "ks"—so "ask" may be pronounced "aks." Further examples are given in Coelho (1991).

There are also syntactical and grammatical differences between West Indian Creole and standard English. For instance, the verb "to be" is commonly omitted in West Indian Creole. "He too stupid" is said for "He is too stupid."

Moreover, there are dialectical differences in plurals, pronouns, and possessives. For instance, in the absence of a quantifier, West Indian Creole marks a plural with a particle—"de book and dem" is said for "some books." The possessive word "mines" is substituted for "mine" (Coelho, 1991). Objective and subjective pronouns are reversed, so one may say "tell she" instead of "tell her" and "him say" instead of "he says."

In addition to dialectical differences, West Indians use many British phrases that differ from American usage. For example, "half-past-two" is said instead of "two-thirty"; "hello" is used to get someone's attention, not necessarily as a greeting, whereas "good night" is a greeting, not a word of departure; and "frock" is used instead of "dress."

Just as teachers have to acclimate themselves to the children's speech, accent, and dialect, the children need time to adjust to American speech and the teachers' idiomatic expressions. A major problem is that West Indian children and their parents do not perceive themselves as needing to learn a new language. Obviously West Indian students have less of a language gap to close than do non-English-speaking students. But if students do not understand that they are to some extent learning a new language, they may not monitor themselves as much as English-as-a-second-language (ESL) students tend to do. As a result, there can be problems with both written and oral language.

In second-language acquisition, a period of silence is needed during which the child listens to or reads the new language without responding. During this time the child is mastering the comprehension of the language. It is important when West Indian children are being assessed linguistically that this be taken into consideration, since children can be erroneously mislabeled as speech-impaired and referred to special education. Adaptation occurs in stages:

1. Initially children speak very little and listen a lot because they are shy and ashamed of their accents.
2. Then they begin to imitate American speech and abandon their West Indian dialect in public. During this stage children are very self-conscious of how they say everything. Only at home do they speak in their native dialect.
3. Finally, they gain confidence and are more accepting of both the American intonation and their West Indian dialect.

The main problem in assessing these students is the absence of an adequate assessment instrument that is culturally and linguistically valid for this population. Thus it is difficult to determine whether a true speech, language, or communication disorder exists. Many of these children are classified as having speech problems when in fact there are simply differences in dialect and pronunciation. But even if these children are classified as having a disorder, they are not always entitled to ESL services, since their language is in essence English. Until scholars recognize West Indian Creole or English Creole as a language with its own grammar and structure, West Indian children are not eligible to receive the services available to bilingual children both in the classroom and in psychoeducational testing. To a large extent, the behaviors and stages observed in West Indian children when making the transition to American speech are similar to those identified in children who are acquiring a second language. The main difference is that while for the most part West Indian children have already mastered the deep language structure, so that they can read and write in English, bilingual immigrant children have not. However, like bilingual children, they still need to acquire the social fluency in the language with respect to pronunciation and accent. Thus the services that these children need are more related to opportunities for conversation and the training of teachers and other educators in West Indian Creole. In other words, the typical ESL curriculum does not fit the needs of the West Indian child, since the purpose of the ESL curriculum is to teach children the basic interpersonal communication skills and cognitive/academic language proficiency: Children usually start from the most basic level, such as learning the alphabet, and receive intensive instruction in vocabulary, grammar, and so forth.

With West Indian children, on the other hand, instruction has to be supplemental rather than intensive. I will refer to this curriculum as "supplemental instruction in the English language" (SIEL). The children are really learning a second dialect rather than a second language. In Canada there is an English-as-a-second-dialect (ESD) program, in which West Indian children learn to speak the vernacular in a program that provides considerable opportunity for oral stimulation. Children are taught to speak more slowly and to represent their thoughts in full sentences. Troike (1968) recommends "guiding [a child] toward an automatic productive control of the mainstream dialect, rather than teaching him from scratch. The goal is to make clear to the child that the choice of dialect is a matter of social appropriateness and expediency rather than one of right or wrong or good or bad" (p. 177). In assessing the West Indian child's speech and language, the focus ought also to be on phonics, since a child who is having difficulty with phonics may have problems with auditory discrimination and certain tense structures, which may create problems with comprehension. This may explain why many West Indian children do well on the comprehension subtests of intelligence tests but do poorly on the comprehension subtests of achievement tests. Comprehension subtests of intelligence tests measure social awareness, social insight, and social judgment in everyday situations. Therefore the average West Indian child, who is quite socially mature, responsible, and moral, will give the correct response as to what is one supposed to do in a particular situation. To effect improvement in this area, one merely has to teach the child the cultural values of the new country by comparing and contrasting them with those of the native land. Achievement tests, on the other hand, usually expect a child to read a passage and then answer questions about it. It measures one's ability to integrate an idea into a whole theme, then break it down before responding to the question. In other words, here a child has to understand the relationship among language, thought, and learning.

Speech and language evaluators must assess whether these children lack an understanding of the basic grammar and deep language structure of English, or whether their difficulty has to do merely with accent or pronunciation. In other words, if a child can read, write, and spell, but speaks ungrammatically—"him say" or "tell she"—then the child is writing and reading in standard English and only using Creole to speak. The child's language here is not related to any intellectual or cognitive deficits, but rather reflects a cultural difference. The child ought to be taught merely that the dialect should not to be used in academic settings, where it may not be acceptable. In other words, children have to learn "to discriminate in which situations each dialect will serve them most effectively" (Coelho, 1976, p. 37).

Soutar-Hynes (1976) recommends that teachers "watch for signs that students are depressed, discouraged, angered" (p. 32). In such cases, the focus must be on identity issues, self-image, the authenticity of the West Indian experience, and the adaptability and sensitivity of teachers to the West Indian culture.

Children who come from the West Indies and who, for various reasons, have not had adequate schooling may need intensive instruction to correct cognitive and academic delays. This issue is discussed in greater detail below. Chapter 15 discusses training implications for speech evaluators and teachers in more depth.

PSYCHOLOGICAL ASSESSMENT

Intelligence Testing: Possible Biases on the WISC-R

Until the 1991–1992 school year, when the Wechsler Intelligence Scale for Children III (WISC-III) was introduced, most West Indian children, like almost all children, were assessed for intellectual development with the Wechsler Intelligence Scale for Children— Revised (WISC-R). So the results of testing West Indian children with the WISC-R will be presented here.

It must be emphasized, however, that neither the WISC-R nor the WISC-III takes West Indian cultural experiences and social customs into consideration. That biases exist on both may cause educators to mislabel West Indian students and misplace them in special education. Cummings (1984) emphasized that "pioneers of mental testing (e.g., Terman, Goddard) regarded the lower IQs of certain immigrant groups as reflecting inferior heredity and were active in eugenics movements designed to restrict immigration in order to protect the U.S. genetic pool from an insidious decline" (p. 66).

What makes West Indian immigrants particularly difficult to assess is that although they technically speak English, they speak various dialects, as discussed earlier in this chapter, and such a dialect may influence an examinee's performance. Figueroa, Sandoval, and Merino (1984) emphasized that "dialects can pose serious problems for psychologists in understanding the full meaning of children's responses" (p. 136). West Indian immigrants are treated as African Americans in the assessment process because most of them are of African heritage, even though the "West Indian family's structure, roles, child rearing and ethnic identity are different from that of American Blacks" (Brice, 1982, p. 123).

Psychologists have found that simply translating these tests is not the answer, since the "content of the tests still remains culture bound" (Gordon, 1980, p. 356). Many items on these tests require information more accessible to white middle-class children and are reflective of white middle-class values.

The following sections examine the possible biases in several questions of various subtests of the WISC-R as they pertain to West Indians. The West Indian educational and personal background, and the implications of such differences for intelligence testing, are also examined. This should help school psychologists more accurately assess the responses of West Indian students on both the verbal and nonverbal subtests.

Verbal Tests

General Information Subtest. Because the General Information subtest is the most culturally biased verbal subtest, it is recommended that it not be included in the standard battery when a foreign student is being tested. The substitute test, Digit Span, should be used, particularly since West Indian children's relative strength is in auditory short-term memory (which is what Digit Span measures). An alternative could be to tabulate two separate IQ scores, one including General Information and one including Digit Span. In this way the child's potential can be determined. Below are examples of culturally biased questions.

Q1. What do you call this finger? [*Show the thumb.*]

In the West Indies the thumb is referred to as "the big finger." Therefore some children may not know the word "thumb."

Q5. How many pennies make a nickel?

The word "nickel" is rarely used in the West Indies, nor is "dime" or "quarter."

Q9. From what animal do we get bacon?

This question assumes that the child knows what bacon is. In the West Indies, the word "bacon" is rarely used. It is best to substitute "pork" for "bacon."

Q11. What are the four seasons of the year?

This should not be asked of a child who has recently arrived from a tropical climate, where there are only two seasons—rain and sun.

Q16. Who invented the electric light bulb?

This question is biased against recently arrived immigrants from less developed countries, where electricity is still a luxury.

Q30. What does turpentine come from?

Fir and pine trees are not grown in tropical climates. West Indian children are at a disadvantage here.

Q12. Who discovered America?

Q17. From what country did America become independent in 1776?

Q19. Name the two countries that border the United States.

Q21. In what continent is Chile?

Q24. How tall is the average American man?

Q27. How far is it from New York to Los Angeles?

These questions are clearly culturally biased, since one cannot expect a recently arrived foreign child to be familiar with American history, American sociology, or questions specifically relevant to an American child's educational experiences.

Similarities Subtest. The Similarities subtest measures verbal abstract reasoning and verbal concept formation. Cummings (1984) points out that when assessing concept formation, evaluators must keep in mind that it is difficult for examinees to know similarities or differences between objects if they have had little or no experience with the objects themselves.

Q4. How are a piano and a guitar alike?

Many children from Third World countries may never have seen or heard a piano. Perhaps "cuatro," another string instrument, could be substituted.

Q5. How are an apple and a banana alike?

Apples are not grown in tropical climates. Perhaps "mango" could be substituted. The important thing here is that a child knows the similarity between different kinds of fruit.

Q9. How are a telephone and a radio alike?

Children who are not exposed to telephones may never have thought about this, and in many Third World countries only the affluent have telephones. Therefore, some children may not have conceptualized in an abstract sense a telephone as it relates to a radio.

Q12. How are a scissors and a copper pan alike?

It may be best to leave out the word "copper." Saying simply "pan" should suffice, since in the West Indies, the term "copper pan" is not a familiar concept.

Comprehension Subtest. In general West Indian children tend to do relatively well on the Comprehension subtest, possibly because of the good moral values in their countries, and also because at an early age children are taught to exercise good social judgment. However, there are biases in the test, as shown in the questions below:

Q1. What is the thing to do when you cut your finger?

A West Indian child may say "put a plaster on it," which is the same as putting on a Band-Aid.

Q6. What is the thing to do when a boy or a girl much smaller than yourself starts to fight with you?

Children from the West Indies may say, "Tell his or her mother or tell the teacher." From a cultural standpoint, this is quite expected and acceptable. For such children to get two points it may be necessary to ask, "Would you fight?" Usually a child will say, "No, it is not good to fight." The important thing to keep in mind is that in such cultures not fighting and telling an adult are the most important things taught to children. In U.S. culture, a child is not necessarily expected to tell an adult.

Q12. Why is it better to give money to a well-known charity than a street beggar?

There are few well-organized charities in the West Indies; therefore, a child will probably say it is better to give to a beggar, because that is the kind thing to do.

Q13. Why is it good to hold elections by secret ballot?

Children originally from nondemocratic societies may have difficulty with this question, since the idea of a secret ballot is foreign to them. The concept is difficult for such children to understand, because in their societies voting is not a private matter.

Q14. In what ways are paperback books better than hard-cover books?

In the West Indies, the term "soft-cover" rather than "paper-back" is used, so it is best to make a substitution of terms with West Indian children. It is important to remember that this subtest is not attempting to assess a child's vocabulary, but rather his or her social awareness.

Nonverbal Subtests

Esquivel (1985) emphasized that "performance scales of standardized intelligence tests appear to have the greatest predictive validity for Limited English Proficient students, and may provide a more accurate estimate of their actual abilities" (p. 119). However, while they may be more accurate assessment tools than the verbal subtests in the assessment of immigrant children, the nonverbal subtests of the WISC-R are also heavily culturally loaded and therefore biased. The Block Design and Object Assembly subtests are biased because most children from rural areas in the West Indies have not had any prior exposure to puzzles and blocks. However, other, more complicated activities that also measure nonverbal abstract reasoning and visual integration (as do the Block Design and Object Assembly subtests, respectively) and are more relevant to the children's cultural experiences are not used instead. The average West Indian boy is very handy; he is often able to help in constructing buildings or making furniture, even though he has had no formal training in these areas. And these tasks are more complicated than putting blocks or puzzles together. But these skills are not measured on a typical Anglo intelligence test. Williams (1980) has emphasized that the very fact that a child can learn certain familiar relationships in his or her own culture shows that he or she can master similar concepts in the school curriculum, so long as the curriculum is related to his or her background experiences.

In addition, on the nonverbal subtests, it is evident that many West Indian examinees pass the higher items after they have already reached their ceiling point (point of discontinuation). It seems as if the children are learning as they go along; thus, lack of familiarity may be why they do not do as well on the earlier items. Unfortunately, by the time they understand how to manipulate the blocks and put the puzzles together, it is time to stop these particular subtests, since they have already reached their ceiling point.

Although these recommended methods of administering the WISC-R may seem quite unconventional and not in keeping with standardized procedures, they constitute a guide for psychologists in tapping the potential of West Indian children. Reporting two IQ scores—one following standard procedures and one taking into consideration the issues raised above—may be the best way to understand these children's strengths and weaknesses. If school psychologists intend to serve children well, they should focus on qualitative rather than quantitative reports that highlight all of the children's past and present cultural experiences.

The Question of Learning Disability versus Mental Retardation versus Educational Deprivation

The question of whether West Indian children are learning-disabled, mentally retarded, or educationally deprived is a major issue raised by educators. Many immigrant children may not have been attending school regularly in their native lands for various reasons; as a result, there may be major gaps in their education. Such children may therefore score several grade levels below their age-appropriate grade placement. Contrary to previous beliefs, intelligence tests tap skills learned both in the home and in the classroom. Thus in most cases it is difficult to determine whether children who were not attending school regularly are truly retarded or even learning-disabled. School psychologists often misclassify these children as learning-disabled or mentally retarded, since they show deficient intellectual functioning on traditional IQ tests in spite of the fact that they score reasonably well on measures of social adaptation. Profiles of mentally retarded and educationally deprived children are similar, since they are both generally flat profiles. The difference is that one is a result of little or no formal education (educational deprivation); the other is a result of continued actual deficits after a child has been formally educated (mental retardation).

In 1973 Mercer found that while an IQ score of less than 70 correlated highly with impairments in adaptive functioning for white children, this was not the case for black children. Mercer found that many black children who did poorly on IQ tests functioned in the average range on measures of social adaptation. The same phenomenon was recorded among West Indian students (Gopaul-McNicol, 1990). Severe academic delays were noted among 56 children recently arrived from the West Indies who were tested at Multicultural Educational and Psychological Services, P.C., in Long Island, New York. The referring school districts thought the children were mentally retarded and would need placement in full-time, self-contained special education classes. But although these children had IQ scores of less than 70, they were average or above in skills of social adaptation. Their daily living skills, coping skills, and interpersonal skills were all for the most part at age-appropriate levels. In fact, many of them, even the intellectually deficient ones, were not only able to take care of basic daily living needs; they were able to cook and sew or do construction work and carpentry, depending on their gender.

Since according to the *Diagnostic and Statistical Manual of Mental Disorders*, third edition, revised (DSM-III-R; American Psychiatric Association, 1987), individuals can be considered mentally retarded only if they are impaired in both social adaptive functioning and intellectual functioning, West Indian children such as these cannot be considered mentally retarded. Yet school psychologists continue to classify such children as mentally retarded without administering a measure of social adaptation. This is especially disturbing since IQ tests are not standardized on West Indian children. Labeling children as mentally retarded on the basis only of an IQ test is not only unethical but also illegal, since the law requires the administration of both measures before a student can be labeled as retarded.

Since these children are not mentally retarded, an examination of their educational experiences in their native countries may shed some light on their scores. Many West Indian children (especially in rural areas) do not attend school regularly, for a variety of reasons touched upon in Chapter 4. During the rainy season floods can block roads, and absenteeism is high as a result. Hurricanes (such as Gilbert and Hugo in 1988 and 1989) have an even more disruptive effect. Survival needs in rural areas also often take precedence over children's education; the children are needed on the farm or in the home. Moreover, it must not be forgotten that several West Indian countries experience continuing political unrest, and this too can interrupt schooling for varying periods of time.

Still another reason some West Indian children are educationally deprived is that many of them cease their formal education after age 11. As explained in Chapters 2 and 4, high school begins at age 12, but in the more developed countries such as Jamaica, Barbados, and Guyana, 60% to 75% of children do not attend high schools because of lack of facilities. On the smaller islands, however, such as St. Kitts and Nevis and St. Martin, where the population is smaller, all children receive a high school education.

It is not surprising that the children who are referred for special education services tend to come from countries (especially Jamaica) where most of the children are not able to attend traditional academic high schools, but instead learn a trade either in a vocational school or on the job—settings in which academic learning is not emphasized. Such children who migrate to the United States at age 14 would not have attended school for about two years. Given an achievement test, they are likely to score significantly below grade and age levels. But it would be a mistake to conclude that they are mentally retarded, when in fact they are educationally deprived. Often these children are able to function in rather mature roles as caretakers for their younger siblings when their parents are at work. As Samuda (1975) points out, "when a two dimensional definition of mental retardation is used, one that takes into consideration not only intellectual performance on tests, but adaptive measures as well, cultural imbalance in classes for the mentally retarded disappears" (p. 11). If a child's social adaptive skills are fine, mental retardation should be ruled out in spite of intellectual deficits.

The question of learning disability versus educational deprivation can best be addressed by examining what constitutes a learning disability. A learning disability is a disorder in one or more of the psychological processes involved in understanding or using language (either spoken or written), which may manifest itself in imperfect ability to listen, speak, read, write, spell, or do math. It does not include learning problems caused by visual handicaps, mental retardation, educational deprivation, or environmental/cultural disadvantages. According to the federal guideline, a learning disability exists when a child does not achieve commensurate with age and ability level in one or more areas after the child has been provided with learning experiences appropriate to age and ability level. Hence a large discrepancy between achievement and ability in one or more of the areas mentioned above constitutes a learning disability. In using a discrepancy between intelligence test scores and achievement test scores to diagnose the existence of a learning disability, one must remember that a child who has not received adequate formal education will inevitably do poorly on achievement tests. School officials must take this into consideration as they assess an educationally deprived child.

Children from the West Indies whose education has been disrupted or truncated for any of the reasons noted above show severe deficiencies in all academic areas, because of significant lack of math and reading skills. But they show little variation between verbal and nonverbal skills. This is significant because a discrepancy of 15 points or more between one's verbal and nonverbal skills is considered to be indicative of a learning disability. Thus most newly arrived West Indian children have profiles indicating educational deprivation, not learning disabilities. Chapter 15 sheds some light on the role that school psychologists can play in assisting West Indian children to acculturate in this society.

Perceptual–Motor Assessment

In administering the Bender–Gestalt test of visual–motor integration to West Indian and West Indian American children, a colleague and I (Gopaul-McNicol & Beckles, 1992) have found that they tend to rotate their Bender designs the first time they are asked to draw them, which has led the school system to label them as neurologically impaired or as having visual–motor deficits. However, when those rotations are pointed out to them, the children are able to correct their errors when asked to redraw the designs. The fact that the children are able to draw them correctly once taught to do so suggests that they perceive the designs differently because of a culturally different interpretation in visual perception, rather than because of visual–motor deficits. We are currently continuing our investigations by assessing via the Bender–Gestalt test the perceptual–motor skills of West Indian American children and West Indian children in the West Indies.

Personality Assessment: Social/Emotional/Cultural

Cultural factors play an important role in personality assessment. At Multicultural Educational and Psychological Services, P.C., there have been several incidents in which children's language was misinterpreted. A classic example was a child who referred to an "eraser" as a "rubber," which is the term used in the West Indies to describe an eraser; the school psychologist said the child was being sexual and promiscuous in the testing situation. Another example was when a West Indian child said, "I can beat him"; the school psychologist did not realize that the child meant "I can win the race," and instead described the child as aggressive and violent.

Recently in Brooklyn, a 6-year-old girl was waiting in line to use the bathroom but was worried that she might urinate before her turn. She approached her teacher while holding her vagina, saying, "My vagina hurt," which was her way of expressing that she needed to urinate badly. The teacher removed her from the line and proceeded to question her about her statement, and several other school officials began barraging the child with questions suggestive of sexual abuse. This led to the allegation that her brother, her father, or both were sexually molesting the child. Not only had the school officials acted inappropriately in interrogating the child (they were supposed to report any suspected cases of sexual abuse to Child Protective Services instead of conducting an investigation themselves), but they did not apologize to the family until legal action was taken against the school district. The family is still traumatized by the experience and in need of long-term, intensive therapy. These are but a few examples of how misinterpretations of West Indian terminology can result in misclassification of children.

In assessing the emotional adjustment of West Indian children in the schools, it is necessary to examine the normal acculturation problems that any immigrant child can experience upon entry into the U.S. school system. In making a healthy adjustment to a new school, immigrant children will first tend to draw on their cultural background as a form of reference, in the same way that kindergarten students draw on their home experiences. Many West Indian children, when they first arrive, are readjusting to their parents after several years of separation, since children are often initially left behind with relatives while the parents get settled and established in this country (see Chapter 2). During this period, children become quite attached to their caretakers, whom they come to know as their parents. When these children are reunited with their natural parents, conflicts arise around such issues as family relations, discipline, and culture. Conflicts also emerge when children are at different adaptation phases than their parents.

Immigrant children can face overwhelming problems in school as they contend with the cultural clash between the norms of their country and the expectations in the host country (Goodstein, 1990). In addition, West Indians typically come from homogeneous nations; they are accustomed neither to racial and ethnic diversity nor to the flagrant racism found in the United States. It is common, therefore, for them to experience confusion and cultural conflict. Chapter 15 explores ways whereby mental health workers can conduct culturological assessment of West Indian clients. In addition, the WICAB (Appendix II) is a tool that can help to determine various stages of acculturation. To gain further information on the overall attitudes of West Indian clients, the West Indian Attitude Survey (Appendix V) or the Immigrant Attitude Survey (Appendix IV) can be used.

Some Questions of Differential Diagnosis

Post-Traumatic Stress Disorder or Emotional Disturbance?

Several of the factors mentioned above and in Chapter 4 as disrupting children's schooling in the West Indies can also have psychological effects on them. Among these factors are natural disasters (e.g., Hurricanes Gilbert and Hugo) and eruptions of political strife (e.g., the invasion of Grenada by the United States in 1983, revolutions in some countries). As a result of events such as these, West Indian children arriving in the United States may well be traumatized. Thomas (1991) has discussed the responses to trauma, given the ages of children. In summarizing the literature, she stated that "the intrusion of memories and thoughts connected to the traumatic event can cause the child to be distracted from an academic task" (p. 5). Thus, compounding the already stressful process of migration, these children are also coping with memories of violence and death. The behaviors exhibited by children in reaction to these stressors can range from withdrawal to aggression. Ronstrom (1989) found that some children became hysterical at loud noises.

Mollica, Wyshak, and Lowelle (1987) have emphasized that in spite of the profound stress these trauma victims experience, many have difficulty articulating their trauma-related symptoms, because the expression of these symptoms significantly increases their emotional distress. The results can be poor academic work, behavioral problems in school, and more difficulty in acculturation. Unfortunately, these behaviors can be misdiagnosed as emotional disturbance. It is vital that school psychologists allow traumatized children the time to acculturate and assist in directing families to supportive centers, where they can receive educational and psychological services to aid in the cultural transition.

Adjustment Disorder or Depression?

Recently, there has been an increase in referrals of West Indian children because of the "depression" noted by school psychologists. Although it is important to be concerned about such symptoms as a lack of interest in social activities, feelings of worthlessness, and depressed mood, it is equally important to bear in mind the DSM-III-R criteria for a diagnosis of depression and the stages of acculturation that immigrant children go through (Chapter 2). Many West Indian children who are referred by the school for therapy because of depressed mood are quite sociable at home and in their communities. In the West Indies, children are taught to be quiet in the classroom; school officials often misinterpret their respect for the classroom setting as withdrawal, shyness, depression, and so forth. Many children say that they are amazed at the liberties that are accorded children in the American classroom. It takes time for them to get used to this liberal, unstructured approach. Simply observing these children on the playground should aid in ruling out shyness and withdrawal.

A more appropriate diagnosis might be adjustment disorder with depressed mood, since many of these children do not continue to show signs of "withdrawal" for more than six months (according to the DSM-III-R, an adjustment disorder cannot have a duration of more than six months). With such patients, as opposed to those with more serious depression, the experience is transient and suicidal ideation (if it exists at all) is likely to be anxiety-producing. Helping clients cope with their anxieties, and providing practical recommendations for dealing with life in the United States, tend to have good results; in most cases, there is no need to resort to pharmacological treatment. In addition, reassuring clients that their symptoms are probably transient and that the therapist can help the clients alleviate them will be useful.

Religious Belief and Mental Illness: Further Questions of Differential Diagnosis

In attempting to understand the causes of mental illness, West Indians rarely invoke psychological explanations. On the contrary, mental illness is attributed to some form of spiritual restlessness meted out to an individual by a vengeful spirit. Many West Indian cultures have a belief in some form of witchcraft that can be worked on someone by an enemy to cause various forms of harm, usually out of envy or a desire for revenge. Folk belief says that when a person is "possessed," a spirit enters the individual's body, and the behavior of the person becomes the behavior of the spirit. It is felt that the more easily influenced a person is, the more likely he or she is to become "possessed." Philippe and Romain (1979) found that females are more likely than males to become "possessed." These folk beliefs are deeply embedded in the culture and can exert a profound influence on people's lives. Many individuals wear a cross as a guard, receive "spiritual baths" (herbal baths with holy water), have a priest or minister bless the home, or even throw salt around the house to protect themselves from these evil forces. These beliefs are accepted by most sectors of society, transcending race, class, age, and gender.

Several of the clients at Multicultural Educational and Psychological Services go to a spiritist while simultaneously seeking psychological help. For example, a woman had sought therapy because her sons had suddenly begun to misbehave "as soon as my mother-in-law had moved into the house." Since her mother-in-law had never accepted her, she attributed the children's misbehavior to her mother-in-law's "evil eye." She talked openly about her suspicions, assuming that I not only understood but would be able to help her in exorcising the children. When I explained my role as a psychologist to her, she was very disappointed that I would not even be able to accompany her to the spiritist. She felt that the problem with her sons was not a psychological one, but a spiritual one. Given the intensity of her belief, I recommended that she seek the counsel of a spiritist first and then resume therapy with me if the negative behaviors of her sons continued after the "bad spirits" were removed from them. She was receptive to this idea and more trusting of the psychological treatment process after she had taken the children to the spiritual healer. It must be pointed out that these beliefs are different from the Haitian voodoo and the Cuban santeria, which are "full blown religious cults with both good and bad magical elements included" (Weidman, 1979, p. 107).

Thus a therapist who hears a parent say, "My child is not conforming because an evil spirit is on him," and then sees the child wearing a chain with a big cross, should neither be alarmed nor think that the family is weird. Similarly, when a woman attributes her husband's infidelity or lack of familial interest to the fact that "someone gave him something to eat that has him tottlebey [stupid]," she is not imagining something, but is expressing a cultural assessment of her husband's behavior. The individual who says, "I see the evil spirit in my house," or "The evil spirit talked to me," is not necessarily hallucinating; nor is the individual who says "God came to me and told me to give up my job, so I did," necessarily delusional.

If mental health professionals are not aware of the folk system, they may misdiagnose a client or devalue or demean folk culturological behaviors. The major point for therapists in assessing psychiatric problems in West Indian families is to try to determine the difference between "being possessed" and true mental illness. When dealing with West Indians, the area of most confusion is in the accurate assessment of schizophrenia, particularly paranoid schizophrenia.

"Possession" or Schizophrenia?

To make a differential diagnosis of "possession" versus schizophrenia, it is first necessary to do a thorough historical assessment of the individual's psychosocial, behavioral, and cognitive functioning. Schizophrenics often exhibit dysfunction in thought, form, perceptions, affect, sense of self, interpersonal functioning, and psychomotor behavior. To be given a diagnosis of schizophrenia, at least two of the following elements must have existed for at least six months: delusions, hallucinations, incoherence or marked loosening of associations, catatonic behavior, or flat or grossly inappropriate affect. In addition, functioning in such areas as work, self-care, and social relations must be markedly low. Schizophrenia is generally treated with antipsychotic drugs, which are useful for eliminating the delusions and hallucinations and alleviating thought disorder.

Many immigrants, while acculturating, may exhibit psychotic symptoms as a result of situational stress. I do not feel qualified, nor do I think it necessary, to enter into the intricacies of folk belief. I will simply say this: It is a pattern of social behavior that has been learned (through constant exposure from childhood onward) and in which people have been conditioned to believe. In other words, it is culturally sanctioned and is even considered to be a spiritually uplifting experience. "Possession is not abnormal, it is normal" (Wittkower, 1964, p. 76). For people who endorse the "spiritual unrest" view, the duration can range from one day to several years. The major point is that West Indians believe a spiritist can remove the evil spirit and free the individual from this "evil force." Therefore, whereas schizophrenics have difficulty eradicating the psychosis, the "possessed" ought not. Treatment approaches discussed in the following chapter should aid in directing therapists how to work with families who maintain these folk beliefs.

"Possession" or Epilepsy?

A state of "possession" (known as "fall-out" by black Americans) also has much in common with epilepsy. As in epilepsy, there are sometimes convulsions, retrograde amnesia ("blackout"), dizziness, and weakness. However, the convulsions are usually seen during the ceremony in which the person is being "depossessed." The common aftereffects and concomitants of the epileptic state—such as incontinent bladder, feelings of exhaustion, and tongue biting—are not evident with the "possessed." This helps to differentiate "spirit possession" from grand mal epilepsy. Philippe and Romain (1979) also found that the responses of "possessed" individuals on the Rorschach psychological test were "far removed from the typical epilepsy profile" (p. 131) because they showed good control over their feelings and normal responses. Moreover, when given an electroencephalogram (a test that helps to determine epilepsy), the "possessed" subjects in Weidman's (1979) study fell within normal limits.

"Possession" or Hysteria?

Hysteria is a more prolonged disease, whereas a "possessed state" is a short-term condition, after which the individual resumes his or her normal personality. Although "possessed" persons show some features of hysteria, "their behavior lacks the marked manipulative overtones so often ascribed to hysterical conditions" (Weidman, 1979, p. 102). A major difference is that hysterics tend to be indifferent to their symptoms of classical conversion, while "possessed" victims are greatly concerned about possible health problems. Lefley (1979) found that the responses of "fall-out" victims reflected little of the impulsivity, lability, and free-flowing emotionality that characterize hysteria. On the contrary, they seemed incapable of emotional responsiveness and tended to deny affectional needs altogether. It was also found that persons who "fall out" cannot be diagnosed as having hysteria of the dissociated type, because while "their consciousness is altered, it is not dissociated in the form of a split personality" (Lefley, 1979, p. 120).

"Possession" or Tourette Syndrome?

Still another source of confusion for clinicians is to differentially diagnose Tourette syndrome from "possession." Like victims of Tourette syndrome, "possessed" persons may shake uncontrollably, grunt, and contort their faces. However, they usually do not use profanity, as is typically done by Tourette patients, and they sometimes maintain an amazingly keen consciousness and awareness of what is going on around them. During the ceremony in which the person is "depossessed," though, a greater loss of consciousness and self-control is noted.

CHAPTER 12

Counseling West Indians

The previous chapter examined cultural issues in assessment and acculturation for the West Indian immigrant. The following two chapters will explore a treatment model for intervening with West Indian families. First, however, it is necessary to examine several issues in this chapter:

1. The concept of psychotherapy for West Indians
2. Family roles as they affect therapy
3. The obligations of children to their parents
4. The process of acculturation
5. The West Indian family in transition
6. The effects of family role changes, disciplinary practices, and housing arrangements on acculturation
7. Religious/folk beliefs and their impact on therapy
8. Language/communication patterns and their impact on acculturation
9. Legal status
10. Intercultural relations
11. Ethnicity
12. The race, gender, and culture of the therapist
13. Therapeutic alliance
14. Resistance—the concepts of time and family secrets

CONCEPT OF PSYCHOTHERAPY FOR WEST INDIANS

West Indians generally do not understand or readily accept either psychotherapy or mental health professionals, as noted in earlier chapters. They tend to seek help as a last resort, and it is usually a child who is identified as the patient. One reason for this reluctance is their lack of exposure to and familiarity with the field of mental health in their home countries. Another reason West Indians have not fully accepted the concept of psychotherapy is that their approach to solving problems is internally oriented. Problems are kept within the family and solved there. The only outsiders who are permitted to intrude are priests or ministers, and the church's role is basically one of providing emotional support and reaffirming the family's belief that God will solve this problem in the right time. Some families in distress may consult spiritists. Such "obeah" practitioners are believed to be able to control evil spirits, which tend to be perceived as the causes of the family troubles (see Chapter 11 and below).

Another impediment to accepting psychotherapy is the social stigma attached to it. The average West Indian believes that a person is either "normal" or "crazy," and only "crazy" people seek psychotherapeutic help. There is little perception of the continuum of behaviors between these two points, or belief that intervention may prevent things from worsening. Also, for West Indians, the causes of "craziness" may be traced to the family, and this may cause a loss of status for the family—something that is extremely important in the West Indian community. There is no parallel to this in American society, where using the services of mental health workers does not reflect nearly as negatively on the family status. For all these reasons, a family is unlikely to seek treatment from mental health workers. Only after all internal family measures and the help of ministers and/or spiritists have failed do the members enter therapy, feeling ashamed and conquered. The therapist must be sensitive to all of these issues if therapy is to be successful.

FAMILY ROLES AS THEY AFFECT THERAPY

In traditional West Indian families, interpersonal relations and interactions are determined primarily by expected roles, duties, and obligations. The role structure is hierarchical and vertical, determined by age and gender. Even if a woman is a professional, her role is primarily one of childrearing and caring for the emotional well-being of her family. Therefore, if a child is having psychological problems, the mother is held accountable. Her most important bond is with her children rather than her husband. The West Indian father is the financial provider and the disciplinarian when the mother "cannot handle the children." His strongest bond is usually with his mother rather than his wife.

Because of the unequal power distribution between parents and children, there is always a need for an intermediary, who may be a well-respected aunt or uncle or even a "parental" child. In West Indian families, the oldest daughter is usually the "parental" child, unless the oldest daughter is considerably younger than the oldest son. The "parental" child is usually the caretaker for the younger ones when the parents are not at home.

The oldest son has many roles. He has to be a source of emotional support to his mother, and he is often an intermediary between his parents, since, should the situation arise, he is expected to defend his mother against his father's abuses. He is also responsible for his younger siblings' educational development and is a financial contributor to his family. The youngest child may, as an adult, be expected to stay at home with the parents. Since this child is the one likely to be the most acculturated to American ways, having migrated at the youngest age, he or she tends to be most vulnerable to familial conflicts resulting from cultural differences.

THE OBLIGATIONS OF CHILDREN TO THEIR PARENTS

American culture emphasizes self-reliance and independence, with high value being placed on one's ability to pull oneself up by one's bootstraps without relying on others. In contrast, West Indian society believes that a person becomes what he or she is through the support of and relationships with many people, especially family members. Therefore, the concept of obligation and reciprocity is crucial, and is an unspoken dictum that everyone understands. This obligation is born of ascribed roles and the understanding of the hierarchical nature of relationships, such as parent–child, employer–employee, and teacher–pupil. This obligatory reciprocity also derives from the sacrifices made by individuals. West Indian immigrant parents are known to work as many as three jobs if that is necessary to give their children an education. One woman illustrated the general attitude when she said to me, "If I have to be a slave in someone's kitchen, I will do it for my son to be a doctor. I do not think about it. I just do it."

In the face of that kind of unflagging support, the greatest obligation children feel is toward their parents. Children feel they can never really repay such a debt, so they give respect to their parents at all costs, even if it means interrupting their own personal lives. It is important for a therapist to understand this obligation, because much difficulty may arise if a therapist tries to help an individual separate or individuate from his or her family. Giving an adolescent assertiveness training without understanding this family ethic can be more problematic than beneficial. Thus it may be more helpful to solicit the help of a significant and close family member, such as an uncle, aunt, or grandparent, who can convey to the parents what the adolescent is experiencing. In other words, detriangulating the most significant people who can aid in the assimilation process should start the ripple effect of change throughout the rest of the family system.

THE PROCESS OF ACCULTURATION

Individuals who immigrate experience two types of cultural transition. The first is a physical transition requiring economic security; employment and educational opportunities; the ability to communicate in the host country; and the ability to understand the social and political differences between it and the native land. The second is cognitive and affective in nature. In this stage individuals have to deal with the psychological pain of "letting go" and assimilating to the new country. In other words, physical arrival in the United States is not the same as emotional arrival. The loss of family, friends, and culture, along with the change in family roles, the hope of "returning home one day," the state of uncertainty, and the expectation that a person has to adapt and acculturate immediately, can lead to stress and dysfunction. Some possible cognitive and affective responses or reactions are grief at the loss of culture, family, friends, and so forth; culture shock and disappointment at the discrepancy between expectation and reality; frustration, anger, and resentment; depression; and acceptance.

Several factors may influence the differences in the rates of acculturation among individuals:

1. Whether they are first-, second-, or third-generation Americans. The longer a family is in the United States, the easier the acculturation process tends to become. However, the number of years in the United States is not an absolute measure, since many immigrants attempt to preserve their culture by freezing traditions.

2. Whether they are children of mixed (West Indian–American) marriages. This can ease the process of acculturation, since one parent is familiar with the workings of American culture.
3. Their language. Fluency in standard English aids in the assimilation process.
4. Their immigration status. Being in the United States legally makes for greater stability and more opportunities for scholarships and higher-paying jobs.
5. Their educational and professional backgrounds. Professional affiliations tend to open doors and help accelerate the acculturation process. Resources such as status and money increase immigrants' esteem among Americans.
6. Their age at the time of migration. The younger an individual, the easier the assimilation process should be.

The ability to acculturate is a crucial indicator of the willingness to change familial roles–a much-needed aspect of cultural assimilation.

THE WEST INDIAN FAMILY IN TRANSITION

West Indian immigration is motivated by opportunities for education and employment, and this move is supported by most family members. As noted in earlier chapters, individuals tend to migrate initially without their children, and often (particularly in the past 10 years) women migrate initially without their husbands. The children are left with relatives (usually grandparents, aunts, or uncles) or friends when both parents migrate. Thrasher and Anderson (1988) reported that of the 30 West Indian families they studied, all of the adult migrants had entered the United States alone, without their spouses or children. In 23 of the families, the children were raised by adults other than the biological parents.

Of particular importance is the fact that in most cases migrants are separated from their families for several years, longer than was anticipated, because of the length of time it takes for them to become eligible to sponsor their families. Contact is maintained by mail and telephone, and migrants usually send goods and money home to their families regularly. Spouses tend to join the immigrants first, followed by the children. Often the children come at different times, not all at once, depending on the immigrants' financial stability. Most immigrants continue to work more than one job in order to bring up members of their extended families. Thus it is not unusual for a West

Indian family to be comprised of the nuclear family, grandparents, aunts, uncles, godparents, and even friends. In a sense, this family structure is multigenerational, with everyone playing a role in disciplining and caring for the children. Thus, when gathering information on a patient, a therapist may have to go to significant others as well as the biological parents. Thrasher and Anderson (1988) have suggested that "when planning and developing social services for this population, viewing the West Indian family from the perspective of the traditional nuclear family, a constellation of biological parents and their children, may not be applicable to this population" (p. 117).

Moreover, because of the prolonged separation of children from their parents, the parents may not be cognizant of many important stages in the children's development. The parents may not be aware of such information as medical inoculation, diseases, and other developmental milestones. Some therapists mistakenly view these parents as "uncaring" because they are ignorant of such important information. Therapists ought not to minimize the effect of the many years of separation on the adjustment of all family members. The years of separation often lead a child to say, "If you love me, why did you leave me for so long?" Parents should be advised that they should plan ahead to take two weeks off to spend with newly arriving children in order to aid in their initial adjustment. This can be planned for by working overtime prior to the family members' arrival, so that no loss of income is necessarily experienced.

Because of the prolonged separation, children may not view the parents as their primary caretakers and may continue to seek the guidance of their grandparents or significant others. A parent who desperately wants to be the primary parent figure again may resent this, resulting in parent–child conflict.

Some of the conflicts center around cultural differences in disciplining, parent's unfamiliarity with age-appropriate behaviors for the typical American children who are their children's counterparts, and parents' unavailability to the children and to school personnel because they have several jobs. It is important to remember that a major aspect of a family in transition is its need for financial security about the fundamental necessities of life—food, shelter, clothing, and (for the West Indian family) home ownership.

Thrasher and Anderson (1988) identified specific school-related problems as the primary source of conflict in the family. These problems included truancy, suspension, fighting, inappropriate class placement, disrespect and verbal abuse to school personnel, discrimination and racism by school personnel, failing grades, poor academic achievement, special education labeling, and discrimination as a result of the West Indian accent.

The re-establishing of the parents' role as the primary authority figures and the transition from one culture to the next are difficult processes, particularly since grandparents or other extended family members often intervene in defense of the children. In addition, parents may feel that the many sacrifices they made and abuses they endured to create a better life for their children are not appreciated. These issues, coupled with such changes as those in school, peers, the environment, weather, and political climate, all exacerbate the tension for the West Indian family.

THE EFFECTS OF FAMILY ROLE CHANGES, DISCIPLINARY PRACTICES, AND HOUSING ARRANGEMENTS ON ACCULTURATION

Changes in family roles have a marked effect on acculturation. A West Indian father may lose his power in decision making and may no longer be the family's sole breadwinner, resulting in his loss of self-esteem. Sharing power with his wife (a discrepancy between U.S. cultural attitudes and those prevailing in his culture of origin) may make him feel that he lacks respect and is a failure as a man. The man experiences even greater displacement if he is unable to obtain employment while his wife can, and he has to remain at home to care for the children. This shift in marital roles may not be as distressing for the man if the woman maintains a traditional perspective on family life. Usually, however, the wife feels more independent and becomes more assertive. If the wife becomes too assertive, challenges his authority, and reminds him who is bringing in the money, the husband may then feel emasculated; often this results in depression. If the man is unable to regain his position of dominance through the major means he was taught—employment—he can panic and attempt to assert his authority in an abusive manner. The ultimate result may be marital separation, caused by the feelings of helplessness and confusion about role change.

Likewise, West Indian women no longer have domestic life as the center of their lives; they are no longer defined mainly by their roles as wives and mothers, but are also employed outside the home. Some even return to school and advance themselves educationally and professionally.

Children also go through periods of role change. They observe their American counterparts and are impressed with their assertiveness and independence; thus they may come to resent their parents' rigid controls, imposed structure, and authoritarian behaviors. They become angry and frustrated about their parents' traditional and "outdated" modes of disciplining them and solving family problems. For example, in an anecdote that highlights the high regard and respect West Indians have for teachers, one West Indian parent on Long Island was so appalled at her son's defiance of a teacher that she publicly scolded and spanked him in the presence of his teacher, actually taking the child's pants down to spank him on the buttocks. The teacher was amazed at such "autocratic measures," claiming, "This was a bit *abusive*." But this is not atypical in the West Indies, even though more acculturated and assimilated immigrant families, who are more familiar with the American social, legal, and political systems, usually do not resort to such measures.

Payne (1989) administered a questionnaire to 499 Barbadians, excluding teachers and child care workers, to determine their views on corporal punishment. This study found that corporal punishment was seen as a means of "teaching right from wrong, lessening the risks of law-breaking when older, [and] training children to grow up in a respectable and decent manner" (p. 397). Payne (1989) also found that the majority (76.5%) endorsed flogging/lashing with a belt or strap as an approved method, with the buttocks most frequently identified as the part of the anatomy to which it should be administered. Slapping with the hand, spanking with a shoe, and hitting the knuckles or palm of the hand with a ruler were approved by 14.4%, 14.2%, and 5.4%, respectively. Burning and scalding (traditional methods used to punish stealing) and lashing out at the child with any object at hand were the forms of corporal punishment most strongly disapproved of. Payne (1989) also noted the types of misconduct for which corporal punishment was considered most appropriate—disrespect to parents/elders, dishonesty, disobedience, stealing, indecent language, violence, deliberate defiance, disregarding the rules of the home/community, and laziness and neglect of chores. Although this study was conducted only in Barbados, "to spare the rod is to spoil the child" is a sentiment shared by most West Indians.

The New York City Department of Planning (1985) reported that an area in Brooklyn with a large West Indian population had a high incidence of suspected child abuse and neglect, ranking fourth out of 59 communities in New York City for maltreatment findings. Thrasher and Anderson (1988) found that physical punishment was used to discipline children in 25 of the 30 families they studied. I found that 84% of the West Indians I surveyed in the West Indies, and 56% of the West Indian immigrants I surveyed in the United States, Britain, and Canada, agreed that spanking is not a form of child abuse. According to Thrasher and Anderson (1988), West Indian parents felt that corporal punishment had been used to guide them into adulthood and they had become successful people. Many such parents express anger, frustration, and confusion that their system of discipline is in conflict with the dominant society and may even lead to allegations of child abuse by people unfamiliar with their cultural mores.

Likewise, housing and sleeping arrangements are in conflict with those of the dominant society. In the West Indies there is no concern about opposite-sex children sleeping in the same bedroom or even in the same bed. It is not unusual to find boys and girls, be they siblings or cousins, sleeping in the same room. In U.S. society, this can be perceived as incestuous, resulting in allegations of sexual abuse.

Mental health practitioners and researchers need to adopt a cross-cultural, dual perspective in conceptualizing and defining child abuse, neglect, and maltreatment in the West Indian communities. In perceiving oneself as abusive, one must accept that a particular act one committed was an abusive one. But this is not the case with most West Indians, especially the recently arrived immigrants. The tasks of the therapist, therefore, are to educate the parents to alternative ways of disciplining their children and to help mitigate the guilt, shame, and cultural conflict that the children experience when they are spanked or reprimanded in the presence of their peers or teachers.

Another area of concern is that children are expected to maintain loyalties to their parents' cultural values. Many West Indian parents expect their children to remain enmeshed with the family, because they are concerned that the children will get too Americanized and "get lost in the system." The family therefore closes its boundaries to the outside world, participating in few cultural events and using few support facilities. This fear of the new environment and a longing for the old one cause the family to isolate itself from the new environment. In attempting to cope, a child may disengage from the family and reject its values. The problem here is that both the child and the family may become vulnerable to an environment that neither fully knows how to negotiate. Children who are caught between conflicts of cultures may develop a negative sense of self and a poor self-image.

The therapist needs to assist youngsters in integrating old values with newly learned ones—in respecting the values of the older generation while forging on and forming their own. An important factor is the sensitivity of the therapist to the preservation of continuities during this fragile process of change. To expect an individual, especially an adult, to become completely Americanized can create anxiety and a feeling of loss of control. It may be beneficial to teach the adolescents to select the best of both cultures and incorporate them into their pool of coping skills. An important factor to note is that the West Indian youths in a study by McKenzie (1986) indicated that counselors who were authority figures seemed indistinguishable from their parents. The caveat, of course, is that such counselors can alienate themselves from youths, because they may appear to be in a conspiratorial relationship with the parents. Therapists must pay close attention to all these factors and familial roles, since these issues are played out in therapy.

RELIGIOUS/FOLK BELIEFS AND THEIR IMPACT ON THERAPY

As I have noted in Chapter 11, few West Indians invoke psychological explanations for mental illness. Rather, mental illness is seen as a form of temporary spiritual unrest meted out to an individual for his or her wrongdoings via a vengeful spirit, evoked by someone who wants to "get back" at him or her. As a result, it is felt that some mental health professionals misdiagnose spiritual problems as personality disorders. Chapter 11 discusses in detail how hallucinations or delusions may be perceived by West Indians.

If an individual's or family's problem is not seen as a medical one, then it is usually categorized as a spiritual one. In such cases, West Indians may first go not to a mental health professional but to an obeah practitioner (a spiritist or a person who practices witchcraft) or a member of the clergy. The obeah practitioner takes into account various aspects of the family situation, such as recent successes and failures; puts them in the context of the cultural belief in spirits; and works out a plan of action according to his or her conclusions.

The healing of an individual usually takes place in a group ceremony known as a seance (although it can be done individually as well). The group is usually comprised of junior spiritual healers, family, and friends. The obeah practitioner who serves as a medium attempts to establish contact with the spirit world in order to determine which evil spirits are creating the person's dysfunction and which good spirits can be enlisted to protect the person. An attempt is made to convince the evil spirits that they should "do good" rather than "do evil." The practitioner will then interpret the spirits' messages for the family, and will prescribe medicinal herbs, ointments, spiritual baths, prayers, and/or massages, all with the goal of helping the individual gain spiritual strength.

Many West Indians believe so strongly in obeah practitioners that merely going to one before the actual exorcism alleviates anxiety. After the exorcism, many experience greater control of their lives and are able to reframe their dysfunctional behaviors more positively. Of course, it is highly probable that a family may only be relaxed enough to trust the therapeutic process after having visited an obeah practitioner. Because of the significant role that obeah practitioners play in the lives of West Indians, regardless of class, race, or gender, research in this area is needed. This is particularly true since a number of therapists from Caribbean backgrounds use them as resources, particularly when patients are deeply involved in this cultural belief. Although this method is quite controversial among traditional psychotherapists, it ought not to be denigrated, since it takes a deep-seated cultural belief strongly into consideration. It is important not to dismiss or ridicule this belief, but rather to help individuals give an explanation for their own dysfunction. Likewise, if a client believes that prescriptions such as herbal baths will be empowering, the practices should not be discouraged. However, the therapist can simultaneously encourage the client to examine alternative choices and to accept some responsibility for his or her situation. Many individuals are simply unaware of alternative interpretations because of their upbringing. The goal should not be to change the belief, but to help clients gain more control over their lives by trusting their own faculties, willpower, and self-discipline. It might be beneficial to place it in the cultural context of the West Indian's general willingness to assume responsibility when things fail.

LANGUAGE COMMUNICATION PATTERNS AND THEIR IMPACT ON ACCULTURATION

Although West Indians do not experience the same sort of language barrier as do non-English-speaking clients, they sometimes encounter difficulty when they speak only West Indian or English Creole. Some older West Indians, such as grandparents, may feel that a counselor does not understand them because of their accent or dialect. When they find themselves having to repeat their answers because of the difficulty the therapist has in understanding them, they tend to become very frustrated and feel that the therapist will not be able to assist them. In other words, they equate the understanding of their language with the understanding of their culture. Those who are already skeptical about the treatment process may use this as an opportunity to terminate therapy.

Of course, the potential cultural barriers are reduced if the therapist can understand the dialect and the nonverbal language. When an individual feels at liberty to express himself or herself, rapport may be established more easily and the possibility of a positive outcome may increase. One grandparent said to me, "Every time I have to say something and think of the standard English way, I lose my train of thought." This brings to mind similar concerns raised by other non-English-speaking clients, justifying the bilingualism of West Indians who speak West Indian Creole.

Some of the main sociocultural factors that influence communication are the following:

1. The generational and age differences within the family make a difference. It is quite common to find older family members speaking only in the dialect, while the younger ones (especially the American-born children) speak only English, even if they understand their grandparents' dialect. Thus, particularly in working with children, it is important to ascertain what language or dialect is spoken at home, in school, and in the community. It is also important to determine in which language each individual can best express emotional and complex matters, and how advanced his or her English vocabulary is.

2. The therapist needs to assess the degree to which a client uses cultural proverbs and nonverbal body language, such as eye contact. Direct eye contact on a continual basis can be perceived as threatening; in the case of an opposite-sex therapist–client relationship (especially if the therapist is a woman), it may even be perceived as a sexual overture.

3. The therapist must be sensitive to topics that a client has difficulty discussing. For instance, in the West Indies discussing sexual matters creates discomfort, especially in older women. Talking about impending death is considered ominous and may be thought to be a sign of bad luck. Such matters should be broached only after a therapeutic alliance has been established.

4. The therapist should ascertain differences in interactive style. For instance, some West Indians (particularly women) may pause, even if they have more to say, in order to get a sense of the impact of what they are saying on the therapist and other family members. The therapist must be careful not to intervene too quickly and by so doing to impede the communicative process.

LEGAL STATUS

To a large extent, the legal status of clients or of schoolchildren determines whether they will feel comfortable opening up to a therapist. The highly publicized case in Long Island, New York, in which a school principal reported two illegal immigrant children, resulting in their fleeing from the school district, is a clear violation of immigration law as it pertains to children in the school system. Although the principal was given a warning because of the inappropriateness of his action, the family was too mistrustful to return the children to the school. Illegal residents tend to draw little attention to themselves, so they may be resistant to therapy, particularly if the therapist has raised their legal status as an issue. Therapists ought to familiarize themselves with the immigration laws (Chapter 2) in order to be of most help to these families.

INTERCULTURAL RELATIONS

Intermarriages are very common among migrants, both interisland (e.g., Jamaican–Trinidadian) and intercultural (e.g., American–West Indian). Some people may intermarry in the hope of balancing out the different characteristics in their own cultures. It is, in fact, likely that the differences are what attract some individuals to each other. However, once in a marital relationship, "the greater the difference between spouses in cultural background, the more difficulty they will have in adjusting to marriage" (McGoldrick, Pearce, & Giordano, 1982, p. 20).

Thus West Indian–American relations may be characterized by more conflicts than West Indian interisland relationships. However, in American–West Indian relations, American men and West Indian women have more successful relationships than West Indian men and American women. The West Indian woman is less threatened by the dominance of the American man, whereas the dominant role that West Indian men play in relationships may prove to be intolerable to the more independent American woman. Of course, it helps to be knowledgeable about differences in cultural belief systems. A person may respond differently when he or she is able to place the spouse's behavior in a wider cultural context, rather than seeing it as a personal assault. However, spouses must also recognize when they are refusing to take responsibility for their actions and instead just asserting, "I am a West Indian; this is the way I am." Friedman (1982) discusses "cultural camouflage" in attempting to explain the tendency of individuals to avoid assuming responsibility for their actions, feelings, and destiny by attributing their behavior to cultural differences or to people who are not sensitive to cultural nuances. Thus individuals may selectively use such differences to justify their position on a particular matter, be it to their spouses or to outsiders.

Interisland relationships may be more or less problematic, depending on the islands. For instance, there may be more conflict when one spouse is from a large island and the other from a small island. In general, however, there is less conflict in interisland marriages than in American–West Indian marriages. Occupational and educational status may, of course, mitigate some of these problems. And people are usually more tolerant of differences in each other when they are not under stress; frustration and anger prevail more readily when people are overwhelmed, and usually at such times, a couple in an intercultural marriage tends to see the problem as a personal one rather than one rooted in cultural differences. Helping the spouses to recognize their behaviors in their own cultural context and to assume responsibility for their "cultural camouflage" is the essence of therapy with such a couple. Learning about each other's responses and interactive styles, as well as gaining an appreciation of cultural variability, is also a requirement in making an intercultural marriage work. This may require a lot of "cultural brokerage" and consciousness raising about one's own cultural values as well as one's spouse's.

ETHNICITY

Racism presents serious problems for the West Indian family in the acculturation process. To begin with, because the West Indies are predominantly black African societies, black West Indians have difficulty endorsing such labels as "minority," "disadvantaged," and "oppressed"; in their cultural experience, flagrant categorical racism was not evident. In the West Indies, lynchings, induced fears, denial of equal opportunity, and racially motivated hate groups are not part of the social fabric. However, West Indian immigrants tend to live in cities such as New York, where the most pernicious elements of racism are subdued and where there are large concentrations of West Indians as well. As a result, there is a built-in support system in the form of a community that aids in the transmission and maintenance of West Indian culture. This is very significant in therapy, because since black West Indians were socialized in a distinctly different world, they do not respond to the U.S. social system in the same manner as African Americans do (see Chapter 8).

In supervising therapists, I have observed the difficulty they have in making distinctions among various black cultural groups. What is hindering this process is the confusion between politics and psychology. While it is understandable that shared loyalties to a political agenda ought to prevail in order to strengthen the political power of all black people, therapeutically one has to address the needs of African West Indians (separate from African Americans) within their psychohistory, psychopolitics, and sociocultural background. Therapists who do not take clients' cultural experiences into account can do more harm than good.

THE RACE, GENDER, AND CULTURE OF THE THERAPIST

Since West Indian family structure is vertical and hierarchical, West Indians as a group "tend to respond best to an older male therapist because this is syntonic with the cultural respect most feel for men and elders" (Brice, 1982, p. 130). Therefore, in working with West Indian families, an inexperienced therapist—especially one who is female and/or young—may do well to solicit the support of a cotherapist who fits this image or of extended family elders who can serve as intermediaries between the therapist and the family. The latter course of action would show that the therapist recognizes and respects the value of elders in the West Indian family and society. A young, female therapist, especially if she is unmarried, may be regarded by the wife as a potential threat and rival for her husband. Male–female team therapy is recommended in such a case. A caveat here is that although West Indian clients may more readily take directives from a male, they may speak more easily to a woman about emotional matters, since women tend to handle such issues in the family. However, both men and women will respect a therapist whom they perceive as a knowledgeable expert.

A therapist of a different race and culture may encounter difficulties in working with West Indian families. A therapist needs to begin by exploring his or her stereotypes, attitudes, and feelings about West Indian immigrants. Although some therapists may have had limited experience with this culture at work or at school, these contacts may have shed little light on the culture of West Indian immigrants or the transition difficulties that they experience. Many therapists simply perceive them as black and dismiss their immigrant status because they speak English, thus denying them the special considerations that are given to most immigrants. Ideally, a West Indian therapist is best. But since many West Indian therapists are not particularly knowledgeable about their own culture, much less that of other islands, a sensitive non-West Indian is preferable to an insensitive West Indian. In general, though, a degree of cultural understanding and similarity helps. A therapist who has experience with immigrant families in general and is aware of West Indian communication patterns (such as the dialect, colloquialisms, and nonverbal expressions) has a greater chance of success in working with West Indian families.

THERAPEUTIC ALLIANCE

In exploring the process in a succesful therapeutic alliance, one must begin by examining the client's expectations of the therapist and vice versa. Once West Indian families have agreed to therapy, they tend to perceive the therapist as an expert, a sort of problem solver who can guide the family in the right direction. The therapist, like the teacher and the medical doctor, is seen as an authority figure and is respected. However, if the therapist does not fulfill the expectations of the family, he or she may lose this respect, and treatment may be terminated. In general, West Indians want a psychotherapist to be active and directive, yet personal, warm, empathetic, and respectful of the family's structure and boundaries. In the initial interview, it is best not simply to wait for the session to flow from the family members, in the hope of observing their interaction; the family may perceive this as indicating a lack of knowledge, confidence, and/or interest. Being active and directive does not mean telling clients what to do or how to live their lives, nor does it mean being too blunt and insensitive; rather, it means taking some initiative and directing the process of the session. For example, the therapist may give some direction as to which family member will speak first; in keeping with the traditional family structure, the husband ought to be addressed first, then the wife, and then the children, according to their ages. If the woman is the one doing most of the talking, the therapist should attempt to assist the man in commenting on her statements. If he is in agreement with his wife, the therapist can mention this to reinforce their unity. At times, the man's silence may be indicative of his quiet strength and the respect he has for his wife's ability to understand the problems of their children. If he disagrees with her, the therapist can point out the validity of different perspectives and different solutions, while attempting to address the problems.

Often a wife may ask the therapist to call her husband and convince him to come in for therapy. This should not automatically be seen as manipulative. West Indian women tend to view this type of request as legitimate, since they perceive authority figures as influential. If this can be done without interfering in the treatment process, it should be; it will help the woman feel that the therapist cares. Since the West Indian man is so powerful in the home, every effort should be made to involve the husband in therapy. Often this can best be done by appealing to his traditional role as head of the family and to his sense of responsibility; he may be more receptive to coming in "for the children's sake." West Indians, especially the men, rarely initiate therapy because of marital problems. Those who do so tend to be more acculturated to American society. Most families who seek help do so because of a child's problem for which a medical doctor was unable to find a physiological cause.

The alliance with children in therapy depends on their ages. With young children, it may be helpful to engage in play and physical contact rather than "talk therapy." With adolescents, it is important to remember that they may have difficulty speaking in front of their parents (especially their fathers), particularly if the topics discussed are drugs, sex, home conflicts, and school problems. It is important and beneficial to hear an adolescent's concerns in private. It is equally important to convince the parents of the importance of doing this. West Indian parents will not automatically respect or even understand this need for confidentiality; for them, confidentiality is neither a right nor a given. But if they believe that part of solving the problem involves the acceptance of this process, they will be more receptive to the therapist's request that they leave the room. Some West Indian parents will nonetheless feel betrayed, because, for the most part, they expect the therapist to assume a parental manner. The goal, of course, should be to help the adolescent to express his or her concerns to the parents and to find ways in which the adolescent and parents can forge a compromise.

In initiating and maintaining a relationship with a West Indian client, it may also help to make home visits, which help to personalize the relationship and to increase trust. For example, the father in a Trinidadian family with whom I was eventually able to establish a wonderful relationship initially refused to come for therapy. When I made a home visit, he told his wife, "She must care"; subsequently, there was no trouble in getting both the father and the other family members to come in for counseling. In later conversations with this gentleman, he told me that he was initially unwilling to come in because he was fearful of the therapeutic process. He said that at home, on his own turf, he felt more safe and more in control, since it was the therapist who was accorded "visiting rights." He felt that he would not have had this initial leverage had he come to the clinic. The first therapeutic/social encounter is crucial if a family is to remain in therapy. The importance of showing deference to the father, and thus acknowledging family hierarchical structure, cannot be emphasized enough.

In establishing a successful therapeutic alliance, a bit of self-disclosure (but not too much) is helpful, since it gives the family some perspective on the therapist. This does not mean telling one's life story or becoming too casual; in response to questions, however, it may be helpful to reveal enough so that the family sees the "human side" of the therapist.

It is important for the family members to feel that they can disagree with the therapist. Since West Indians tend to confer respect on a therapist once trust has been established, it is difficult for them to express anger or criticism toward the therapist, especially if he or she has been helpful in resolving some family conflicts (because obligation was thus incurred). The therapist must be responsive to nonverbal cues, such as changes in facial expression, sudden silence, or changes in vocal inflection, all of which may be indirect indicators that someone is angry or not in agreement and is trying to suppress his or her feelings. Such suppression of feelings may also be noted in lower-status individuals toward higher-status individuals in the family. It is likely that this reluctance to open up may result in the family's terminating treatment without telling the therapist why.

Another issue is the use of first names. With West Indian families, it is best to address adults as "Mr." or "Mrs." and to be addressed similarly by them in return. Children can be addressed by their first names.

Likewise, dressing in a "professional" manner reflects respect for the clients. In the West Indian community, professional people are expected to dress in keeping with their station in life; formal dressing distinguishes professionals from nonprofessionals.

Yet another important matter to note is that it is not unusual for West Indian families to give gifts to the therapist (just as they give gifts to teachers) and to send cards even after treatment is terminated. Accepting such gifts should not be construed as "unprofessional." The message being conveyed is that a good relationship is a long-lasting one that should be treasured. Refusing such a gift, given as a token of gratitude for assisting the family in a time of crisis, can be seen as insulting. Besides, the gift is not given instead of monetary payment for the therapist's services.

In general, to establish a successful therapeutic alliance, it is necessary to explore the cultural strengths of the family; to demonstrate a caring attitude; and to be directive, warm, and "human," but not too friendly. In addition, it is best to be flexible with respect to home visits.

RESISTANCE—THE CONCEPTS OF TIME AND FAMILY SECRETS

In spite of all attempts to foster a therapeutic alliance, many West Indian families remain resistant to therapy. Two factors in particular play a part in resistance with the West Indian family—the concepts of time and family secrets.

Lack of observance of scheduled appointment times is a major concern in therapy with West Indian families, who in a social sense endorse the adages "Any time is West Indian time" or "Better late than never." Socially, West Indians tend to visit friends at any time without an invitation or without calling. Because of the informality of West Indians, many clients miss appointments or appear at unscheduled times, expecting to be seen. They also give priority to job demands and will not sacrifice work for therapy, because they take very seriously the aphorism that "time is money." However, such behavior does not necessarily reflect resistance to therapy. One must keep in mind that one of the major reasons why West Indians migrate is to seek a better life, be it educational or occupational. And as has been mentioned in many prior contexts, it is typical for adults to hold at least two jobs. Therefore, a therapist may have to be flexible in scheduling treatment so that therapy does not interfere with educational or work opportunities. If treatment results in the loss of wages, the family or individual may become resistant and resentful.

Although West Indians may appear to be engaging socially, sharing real family secrets is a different issue. Secrets are to be kept within the family unit. Every child is told very early, "Do not put our business on the street." Therefore, discussing personal and family issues openly and freely with a stranger is often very difficult. West Indians also tend to deny family problems because they believe there is nothing that they cannot solve themselves within the family. They indulge in much circumlocution, especially in the initial stages of therapy. Thus, unless the therapist has clinical evidence that a secret is hindering the therapeutic process, the therapist is advised (particularly in the initial stages) to proceed on the assumption that the secret may merely be a maneuver to keep boundaries in place. Pushing the family to tell the secret too early in therapy may provoke mistrust and resistance, thus jeopardizing the therapist's position.

Major Treatment Approaches in Counseling the Culturally Different

With the continued increase of immigrants entering the United States from various cultures, researchers, teachers, and mental health workers are faced with the challenge of acquiring a working knowledge of each group's customs, norms, history, and so forth. Although it is impossible for any therapist to understand the traditions, values, and languages of all immigrant groups, a therapist (in spite of his or her limited knowledge) may be guided by conceptual, operational principles that can be implemented across diverse groups and circumstances. This chapter explores several treatment techniques that can apply to immigrants, with particular attention to the works of Sue, Pedersen, Helms, and Dillard (emphasis on culture—*multicultural*); Lazarus, Bowen, and Minuchin (different modes of therapy—*multimodal*, educational, structural); and Boyd-Franklin (*multisystems*).

MULTICULTURAL COUNSELING

Multicultural counseling has become a popular concept among practitioners and researchers, because it is a way to acknowledge cultural diversity between therapist and client. Dillard (1983) includes in the definition of "culture" a shared belief system, behavioral styles, symbols, and attitudes within a social group. Assimilating to a particular culture is a slow process that involves adopting some dominant social and cultural norms, and possibly losing a sense of cultural identity with one's original culture. In attempting to conduct multicultural counseling, the goal must be to help the culturally different client to adapt to or reshape his or her psychosocial environment (Dillard, 1983).

Sue (1981) has examined the underlying principles in attempting to counsel the culturally different. His major point is the importance of the therapist's being knowledgeable about the client's culture and lifestyle in order to provide culturally responsive forms of treatment. Taking the role of culture and culturally relevant techniques into consideration in psychotherapy is one of the most difficult challenges facing the mental health profession. The problem is exacerbated when therapists overgeneralize what they have learned or act on insufficient knowledge. Sue and Zane (1987) emphasize that changes have to do with the process of "match or fit." Treatment should match or fit the cultural lifestyles or experiences of clients, in order to prevent premature termination and underutilization of services and ultimately to result in positive outcomes. In general, Sue and Zane stress the need for multicultural centers, where continuing educational programs on cultural issues should be made available, as well as legal, social service, and language programs; such centers are particularly necessary in communities where large ethnic or culturally different groups exist. Of course, the authors recognize that while cultural knowledge may increase therapist credibility, it can be quite irrelevant to positive therapeutic outcomes if the knowledge is not transformed into concrete, effective strategies. Thus knowledge of the culture; the formulation of culturally relevant, consistent (yet non-cookbook-type) strategies; credibility (the client's perception of the therapist as an effective and trustworthy helper); and "giving" (the client's perception that something has been received from the therapeutic encounter) are all important and necessary in providing more adequate service to the culturally different.

Implicit in cross-cultural psychology is the notion of biculturalism. Many theorists view biculturalism as the healthiest identity resolution in the United States, although some view it as an abandonment of one's cultural heritage. Pedersen (1985) sees biculturalism as an addition to one's original heritage and examines the process by which cultural identity develops, since intercultural interactions influence one's behavior. Helms (1985) outlines the three stages of cultural identity.

The first stage, the pre-encounter stage, is the phase before the individual's cultural awakening. In this stage, the individual is so enmeshed in the Eurocentric view that he or she idealizes white culture while degrading his or her own culture of origin. The affective state associated with the first stage is both poor individual and group self-esteem.

The second stage, the transitional phase, occurs when the individual comes to realize his or her lack of absolute acceptance by the white world. The individual goes through a period of withdrawal and cultural reassessment, ultimately deciding to become a member of his or her own cultural group. Dillard (1983) points out that in this stage the individual sees his or her cultural system as superior to other cultural systems. It is a stage of ethnocentrism. The affective state is one of euphoria, a sort of spiritual rebirth, as the individual tries to identify with his or her culture of origin. However, there is also confusion and sadness as the individual realizes that there has been some loss of cultural identity, since he or she cannot identify with *all* the values of the original culture.

The final or transcendent stage occurs when the person becomes bicultural and uses the experiences from both cultural groups that best fit his or her own circumstances. In this stage, the individual is more accepting of the flaws in both cultures and does not idealize either group. Affect is more temperate, and an identity resolution is experienced. Interpersonal relations are not limited by race, culture, gender, and so forth; a broader perspective is endorsed. Self-esteem is improved. This stage is attained after the person experiences an identity transformation, via personal readiness and educational and cultural socialization experiences requiring flexibility. Recommendations for therapists on how to best treat individuals in these various stages are discussed in Chapter 14.

MULTIMODAL THERAPY

The aim of multimodal therapy is to reduce psychological discomfort and promote individual growth by recognizing that few, if any, problems have a single cause or a single cure. Instead, the disquietude of people is multilayered and requires a holistic understanding. Lazarus (1976) dissected human personality by examining the interaction among multiple modalities—behavior, affect, sensations, images, cognitions, interpersonal, and biological (BASIC IB). To make the acronym more compelling—BASIC ID—the biological modality was originally labeled "D" for "drugs," although it actually includes the full range of medical interventions (e.g., nutrition, hygiene, exercise, medication). The multimodal assessment focuses on the behaviors that get in the way of one's happiness and how one *behaves* when one feels (*affect*) a certain way, as well as what the *sensations* (e.g., aches and pains) are and what bearings these sensations have on behavior and feelings. In addition, the goal is to examine how one perceives one's body and self-*image*, how one's *cognitions* affect one's emotions, and what one's intellectual interests are. Who the most important people in one's life (*interpersonal*) are and what they are doing to one are also explored. Moreover, the focus is on any concerns one has about the state of one's health and the *drugs* or medication that one uses.

Educational Approach

In Bowen's (1978) systems therapy, the therapist is portrayed as a teacher who utilizes an educational approach to therapy. This approach recognizes the value of education and research in self-change. Bowen, also an advocate of the multigenerational perspective, focuses on transgenerational patterns. Thus, what has occurred in the past and what the older generation feels about it are important in Bowenian therapy. One goal of therapy is to increase differentiation of individuals within their families. Another goal is to decrease individual anxiety and emotional reactivity by diverting the focus from the "identified patient" to past and present family members. Doing this permits the individual to think clearly and avoids the need for triangulation or emotional cutoff, which Bowen believes occurs when anxiety is high. He engages more often in couples therapy than in family therapy, but he encourages spouses to work on their relationships with their families of origin, based on the assumption that unresolved issues with one's original family affect current family relations. Therapy constitutes a cognitive re-encounter with one's past as it is represented in one's present life. The focus is on facts and patterns, not feelings. Bowen also establishes leverage within the family system by discovering the most likely entry point (the person most capable of change, i.e., the least resistant family member). He then uses this least resistant, most motivated member to deal with the resistance of other family members.

Structural Approach

The structural approach to family therapy is mainly associated with Minuchin (1974). The focus is mainly on boundaries, the patterns of the family, and the relationship between the family system and its wider ecological environment. An individual's symptoms are perceived as stemming from a family's failure to accommodate its structure to the changing developmental and environmental requirements. These dysfunctional reactions to stress create problems that manifest themselves in family interrelations. The responsibility for change rests primarily on the therapist, who utilizes three strategies—challenging the symptom, challenging the family structure, and challenging the family reality. The therapist must negotiate the family boundaries in such a manner as to be given the power to be therapeutic. These boundary issues incorporate the concepts of "enmeshment" (in which some or all of the family boundaries are relatively undifferentiated or permeable) and "disengagement" (in which family members behave in a nonchalant manner since they have little to do with one another, because family boundaries are very rigid and impermeable). Although most families fall within the normal range, Boyd-Franklin (1989) has stated that the cultural norm among black families tends to fall within the enmeshed range.

Aponte (1976), one of Minuchin's colleagues, discusses the issue of the power of some family members, who may or may not be in therapy with the identified patient. Aponte emphasizes that even if one conducts several therapy sessions with the identified patient and other family members, change may be sabotaged because of a powerful family member who did not become involved in the therapeutic process. This powerful member may influence the other members to terminate or continue treatment. Thus the therapist is advised to explore as early as possible who the truly powerful family members are. The therapist needs to find out such information as whom the client goes to before making a decision, which family member has the final say on most matters, whom the client listens to most in the family, and who tends to disagree most with the client's decisions. These questions can help in identifying the powerful figure who needs to be more directly involved in therapy.

MULTISYSTEMS APPROACH

Boyd-Franklin (1989) has emphasized that effective therapy with black families requires from the therapist a flexibility that allows him or her to draw from different systems theories and incorporate them into an overall treatment plan. It also requires the therapist to intervene at a variety of systems levels, such as individual, family, extended family, church, and community and social services. Boyd-Franklin's multisystems approach has been quite challenging to traditional theories in the field of mental health. Many clinicians feel that working with social service agencies and churches is the task of a social worker and not a clinician. Many therapists also feel overwhelmed by the complexity of this multisystems model. However, in working with black families, establishing rapport and building credibility are necessary and may involve intervening in numerous systems and at many levels. This model was built on Minuchin and associates' (Minuchin, Montalvo, Guerney, Rosman, & Schumer, 1967) and Minuchin's (1974) structural family systems model; Aponte's (1976) ecostructural approach (Aponte & Van Deusen, 1981); and the ecological approach of a number of theorists, such as Auerswald (1968), Bronfenbrenner (1977), Falicov (1988), Hartman (1978), Hartman and Laird (1983), and Holman (1983).

The multisystems approach, which comprises two main axes, is based on a concept of circularity rather than one of linearity; in this respect, it differs from most treatment approaches. Axis I, the treatment process, is composed of the basic components of the therapeutic process: joining, engaging, assessing, problem solving, and interventions designed to restructure and change family systems. Each component can recur throughout the treatment process at all systems levels. Axis II is made up of the multiple levels at which the therapist can provide treatment, such as individual, family, extended family, nonblood kin and friends, church, community, social service agencies, and other outside systems.

THE INTEGRATION OF THE THREE APPROACHES WITH WEST INDIAN FAMILIES

The three approaches—multicultural, multimodal, and multisystems—can be effectively combined in a treatment process in working with West Indian immigrant families. I discuss this treatment model at length in the next chapter. First, however, I point out the specific relevance of the works discussed above to therapy with West Indian families, as well as certain variations or additions that will be needed.

Sue's (1981) major point is the importance of the therapist's being knowledgeable about the client's culture and lifestyle. The critical roles of the therapist's credibility in treatment and of the therapist's methods are also highlighted. The concept of "giving" is also an important factor in the client's trusting the therapeutic process. Sue's suggestions and techniques are all relevant to West Indian families at various stages of therapy.

Helms's (1985) three-stage model of cultural identity development—the pre-encounter stage, the transitional stage, and the transcendent stage—is applicable to the process of acculturation for West Indians.

Lazarus's (1976) multimodal approach, emphasizing BASIC-ID—behavior, affect, sensations, images, cognitions, interpersonal, and drugs—can be quite beneficial in assisting in the acculturation process. For many families, the migration process is full of stress because of the many adjustments that have to be made in the host country. This holistic approach to mitigating these stressors can be very effective with West Indian families.

Bowen's (1978) systems therapy, in which the therapist is portrayed as a teacher, is quite compatible with the West Indian perspective on securing and accepting help. Bowen's multigenerational perspective can also be quite fruitful, since unresolved issues with one's original family may affect current family relations. With West Indian families, examining events that occurred as many as three generations ago may help the therapist see transgenerational patterns that affect current functioning. Moreover, since West Indian families tend to be highly enmeshed, Bowen's technique of increasing individual differentiation is necessary near the midphase of the treatment process. In addition, Bowen's focus on facts and patterns rather than feelings may prove to be less threatening in the initial stages, while Lazarus's focus on feelings (affect) may be useful in the middle and end phases of therapy. Although some theorists (Brice, 1982; McKenzie, 1986; Sewell-Coker, Hamilton-Collins, & Fein, 1985; Thrasher & Anderson, 1988) agree that the best approach to working with West Indians is to de-emphasize emotion, because "it is likely that questions aimed at feelings may reach a dead end" (Brice, 1982, p. 131), it is my experience that once West Indian clients (including men) trust the therapist, the affective dimension can be addressed. This is best dealt with in the middle to end phases of therapy, since in the initial stages there seems to be some sort of covert agreement by all family members to conceal their feelings. It must be pointed out, though, that because of West Indians' resistance to (or, rather, lack of understanding of) the therapeutic process, therapy tends to be short-term; as a result, emotional issues are not always dealt with before the clients terminate.

Minuchin's (1974) structural approach to family therapy is also relevant for West Indians, since it emphasizes that an individual's symptoms can be attributed to a family's failure to accommodate its structure to changing developmental and environmental requirements. Like many immigrants, West Indians have difficulty "letting go" and adopting the concept of biculturalism. Many of them live in the United States without becoming citizens or celebrating American holidays. Had it not been for the children, many West Indian parents might have continued quite contentedly living between two worlds. Minuchin's approaches of challenging the family structure, challenging family reality, and renegotiating family boundaries are all helpful techniques in addressing the issue of enmeshment and power. Aponte's (1976) approach of bringing the most powerful family member into therapy is also needed in working with West Indians, because it is usually the father who is absent from therapy, and in most cases he is the most powerful person in the home.

Boyd-Franklin's (1989) multisystems approach—individual, family, extended family, church, community, and social services—provides a flexible set of guidelines for intervention with West Indian immigrants. Empowering families, establishing rapport, and building credibility are more easily achieved by using multiple systems and intervening at many levels. Some important additions to this model in working with West Indian families are the school/educational system and the legal system as it applies to immigrant status.

CHAPTER 14

The Multicultural/ Multimodal/Multisystems Approach to the Treatment of West Indian Families

While the mental health field has begun to recognize the need for flexibility in working with the ethnic and culturally different, little research has been done on treatment approaches with English-speaking West Indian American clients. The therapist who works with West Indian American clients, as with most culturally different groups, must be willing to be flexible and draw from the work of a variety of cross-cultural theorists and various therapeutic modalities.

The multicultural/multimodal/multisystems approach—hereafter referred to as the Multi-CMS approach—was developed from my own clinical experiences in both the United States and the West Indies, where I conduct seminars and workshops for educational and mental health professionals who work with this population. After interviewing 873 West Indians in the West Indies, the United States, Britain, and Canada, and after visiting 15 West Indian islands, where I observed and worked with children both in school and at home, I believe that this comprehensive approach to therapy is the most effective in working with West Indian immigrants. This does not mean that a therapist should be rigidly constrained and not develop his or her own personal style and mode of treatment. It is my hope that the theoretical framework presented here will serve as a source of information for those who lack the necessary knowledge, as a reminder for those who unintentionally forget, and as a reinforcement for those who sincerely attempt to understand and accept West Indian clients. Although this model is discussed primarily in relation to West Indians, it has direct relevance to other cultural groups.

Unlike many treatment approaches, which are based on linear models, the Multi-CMS approach (like Boyd-Franklin's [1989] multisystems approach) is based on the concept of circularity; it consists of four phases, and each component of each phase can recur repeatedly at various levels throughout the treatment process. The therapist must be flexible enough to intervene at whatever level is needed at whichever phase in therapy. With this in mind, the flow of treatment for the Multi-CMS approach is as follows:

Phase I. Assessment process
    Step 1. Initial assessment
        A. Explaining the process
        B. Establishing trust
    Step 2. Gathering information
    Step 3. Determining the stage of acculturation
    Step 4. Outlining the goals
Phase II. Educational treatment process
Phase III. Psychological treatment process
Phase IV. Empowerment treatment process

PHASE I. ASSESSMENT PROCESS

Step 1. Initial Assessment

The initial assessment stage, which occurs in the first therapy session, is divided into two phases: (1) explaining the process and (2) establishing trust. For the reasons described in Chapter 12, many West Indians are initially resistant to therapy. Most West Indians who enter therapy are referred by school personnel or child protective services. In an effort to establish a relationship, the therapist must explain the therapeutic process as clearly as possible, because many West Indians view psychotherapy as a visit to a medical doctor. Many do not understand how merely talking about one's problem can bring about an actual change. Many believe that therapy will last for only one session and that only the identified patient (in most cases, a child) will be involved. Furthermore, most families referred by child protective services do not believe they should be there; as far as they are concerned, their forms of discipline are appropriate. To the therapist this attitude may appear defensive and resistant, but from the clients' perspective it is sensible. Most people in their countries of origin discipline their children with corporal punishment. Therefore it is important that the therapist not belittle the disciplinary measures they have used in the past, but rather explain that there are cultural differences between the West Indies and the United States in practically every aspect of life.

At this juncture the process of psychotherapy can be explained. Highlighting how the parents will be taught alternative ways of disciplining their children and other gains that will come from therapy must be done from the outset. It is also necessary to explain that a therapist works with "normal, healthy" people who are simply experiencing adjustment difficulties, not just "crazy" people, as many West Indians tend to believe. The therapist should explain that therapy usually lasts approximately one hour (although the initial session can take as long as two hours), and that at times it may be necessary to see the entire family, not only the identified patient. Many families are not aware that they are expected to pay and become even more angry when told this. This is because they know that a visit to a doctor involves a one-time payment, and that informal social support in the community is usually free. Examining their health insurance or any other medical plans can alleviate some of the anxiety regarding full payment. The first 15 minutes of therapy involve clearing up misconceptions about psychotherapy and explaining the process of treatment. Questions can include the following:

1. _Why are you here?_ Given the clients' response, the therapist should help alleviate any guilt or anger via empathetic understanding. If their understanding of why they are there is different from that of the referral source, the therapist should mention the discrepancy only if it will not hurt the therapeutic alliance. If there is denial on the clients' part, it can be addressed later in the session.
2. _Were you ever in therapy before?_ If they were not, the therapist should explain the therapeutic process.
3. _What are your thoughts about a psychotherapist or about psychotherapy?_ The therapist should address any misconceptions or anger about being in therapy.
4. _What do you think you can gain from therapy?_ In other words,

what do the clients want the therapist to address immediately? Addressing what the family views as most pressing will help to build the therapist's credibility, as well as empower the family.

It may also be important to note the following:

1. The seating arrangement of family members—who sits next to whom?
2. Who is the powerful figure in the family?
3. Who speaks on behalf of the family?
4. Are the children allowed to speak?
5. What significant family members are missing?

The next stage of this initial assessment process is the establishment of trust. This can be done through Sue's concepts of credibility and giving. "Credibility," according to Sue and Zane (1987), refers to the client's perception of the therapist as an effective and trustworthy helper. Credibility can be ascribed or achieved. "Giving" is the client's perception that something has been gained from the therapeutic encounter. For West Indians, a therapist's credibility depends at least initially on his or her ascribed status in keeping with cultural factors: age, gender, and education. In West Indian culture, the youth is subordinate to the elder, the female to the male, and the less educated individual to the more educated authority figure. A lack of ascribed credibility may be the main reason West Indian clients resist therapy. Credibility can also be achieved (instead of ascribed) through the therapist's culturally relevant techniques, skills, and empathetic understanding. A lack of achieved credibility may be the reason clients terminate therapy prematurely. This is why the first session is so important in establishing credibility. West Indian clients will trust and view the therapist as more credible if he or she conceptualizes the problem in a manner consistent with their cultural experiences and beliefs. Thus it may be more beneficial, for example, if the therapist appears to understand how a parent can spank a child. Conversely, a therapist who tells a child to be very assertive to his or her parents may lose credibility.

It is important to remember that with this model, the assessment process (and the therapeutic process) is ongoing and cyclic. Another important factor is that from the inception of therapy, the therapist is engaging in some form of intervention, some sort of problem solving; if this is effective, the client's fears, misconceptions, and confusion begin to be alleviated minutes into the first session.

Step 2. Gathering Information

In the second stage of the assessment process, the WICAB (Appendix II) may prove beneficial. Because it is very detailed, it may be necessary to focus only on the areas that are relevant to the client's or family's problems. Alternatively, it can serve as a guide in determining where the problem areas for the family are.

Boyd-Franklin (1989) mentions that information gathering on black families often occurs later in the treatment process. She attributes this to the process of building trust, which must be established before extensive information gathering can take place. Although this may also be applicable to some West Indian families, most want to get on with whatever is necessary so that they can be finished with therapy. Therefore, the therapist must determine whether the family is ready to engage in data collecting in the first session. It is important to keep in mind that with West Indians, a therapist can establish credibility in the first few minutes of the first session merely through ascribed status. The therapist ought to be aware that copious note taking can be quite intimidating and distracting, since families may feel the therapist is not paying attention.

The genogram, a tool derived from anthropology but quite commonly used in psychology, is a sort of family tree. This can prove to be quite useful to the therapist working with West Indian families because of the many family members and friends who are directly or indirectly involved. If nothing else, it will allow the individual or family to visually represent support systems. However, as discussed in Chapters 4 and 11, West Indians, because of the nature of their countries' educational systems, use auditory learning modes better than visual ones. Therefore the use of drawings and maps, such as the genogram, may not necessarily result in engaging the family. It can be equally beneficial simply to record the information without the use of a tree, using such questions as "Who raised you?" and "Whom did you live with prior to coming to the United States?" Once a picture has been drawn, the therapist can encourage the family to bring in some or all of the family members who have an impact on the life of the identified patient.

Step 3. Determining the Stage of Acculturation

It is important to keep in mind that not all families are really in need of therapy because of acculturation difficulties. Therapists should be careful not to overinterpret cultural issues, since many families negotiate the acculturation process with little difficulty. Some families need therapy for the same reasons American families need therapy—for instance, the teenage rebellion typically found in any culture. However, with immigrant families, difficulties in acculturation can be a major factor contributing to their family problems. The discussion of Helms's (1985) three stages of acculturation in Chapter 13 is relevant to West Indian transitional conflict. Determining whether there is any transitional conflict is a key to helping immigrant families. The WICAB contains questions the therapist can ask to determine the stage of acculturation the individual or family is in and how they have dealt thus far with the vicissitudes of the prior stages. The answers to these questions will help the therapist determine the goals for therapy.

Step 4. Outlining the Goals

In establishing credibility, it is necessary, before the end of the first session, to outline very briefly what the individual or family will gain; that is, the goals of therapy should be highlighted. If there is a discrepancy between a client's goals and the therapist's, the therapist's credibility will be diminished. As a matter of practice, at the end of every session, it is wise to re-evaluate progress and see whether the goals are being accomplished. Of course, even as the goals are being outlined, therapy can begin. Here again is a reminder that one advantage of this comprehensive model is that therapy can begin even while assessment is still in progress, because of the cyclical nature of this treatment approach.

PHASE II. EDUCATIONAL TREATMENT PROCESS

In working with immigrant families, much of the therapy may be educational in nature, since many adjustment difficulties may be the results of cultural differences or a lack of knowledge about the U.S. educational, social, legal, and political systems. If the assessment process reveals that the family members lack knowledge about these basic systems, which they have to deal with every day, they may have to be educated about them. My colleagues and I (Gopaul-McNicol et al., 1991) explore basic educational and social issues of which immigrant families need to be aware and the facilities that are available to help them in the process of adjustment.

A colleague and I (Thomas & Gopaul-McNicol, 1991) have examined immigrants' understanding of the American school system, particularly the special education process (a concept foreign to West Indian families). The term "special education" is not used in the West

Indies. In fact, in the West Indies, children who are performing well below or well above grade level are either held back another year or moved up a grade. Therefore, many families believe that special education may be best for their children "because they are receiving extra help," and that the school "is kind" to provide this supplementary service. We have examined the factors that affect the immigrant child's adjustment in school, the procedures for placing children in special education, the symptoms of handicapping conditions, and the parents' role in special education.

In regard to the legal system, the next treatment stage for clients who are in this country illegally is to educate and empower them. This may involve such things as helping them find an immigration attorney, or explaining their rights with respect to their children's education. This means that the therapist must know the various systems, be willing to establish contact with the different service providers in these systems, and if necessary include these providers in therapy sessions. This stage of therapy may also involve a lot of homework, such as reading (bibliotherapy), to gain an understanding of the various systems. As can be seen, effective therapy with West Indian families requires flexibility, the use of a circular model, and even the removal of some traditional boundaries. Therapists must be willing to explore the impact of the educational, social, legal, political, and social conditions of the families they treat. To attempt to treat these families without addressing these systems may impair the therapist's credibility.

If the assessment shows that a black West Indian immigrant child is in the pre-encounter stage described in Chapter 13, then the therapist can expect him or her to endorse a Eurocentric view and to feel ashamed of his or her parents, accent, clothes, foods, and so forth. The parents, in turn, may feel rejected, frustrated, angry, and confused. In this stage, therapy has to focus on both the parents and the child. Parents must be taught the social and emotional adjustment stages that children go through. The goal of therapy is still educational at this point, since the therapist needs to assist the West Indian parents in understanding the following:

1. The causes of childhood misbehavior, and the principles and concepts underlying the social learning of such behavior.
2. The cultural differences in values and discipline as they affect their child's adjustment.
3. The emotional stress and fears that emerge in a child as a result of migration and adjustment to a new family, and the difference between an emotional disturbance and cultural adjustment.
4. The differences in the school structure and school expectations.

5. The criteria used by the school system in placing children in special programs, and their parental rights in such a case.
6. How the parents can build positive self-esteem and self-discipline in their child via a home study program, so that the child will be empowered to maintain a positive self-image in this race-conscious society.
7. How to communicate more effectively with their child, and how to be critical without affecting their child's self-esteem.
8. The impact of peer pressure and how it can be monitored.

Chapter 15 sheds some light on how therapists can train parents in these areas.

In this preencounter stage, therapy for the black West Indian immigrant child should be both educational and psychological, since the child ought to be taught the following:

1. To understand the sociocultural differences between his or her native country and the United States (educational).
2. To cope with peer taunts about accent, mode of dressing, foods, family, and so forth (psychological).
3. To communicate more effectively with his or her family (educational and psychological).
4. To acquire the social skills and assertiveness skills needed (psychological).
5. To improve study skills and to understand cultural differences in test taking, school structure, school expectations, and language factors (educational).
6. To cope with the emotional stress and fears that come with migration (psychological).
7. To understand the psychology of being black in American society (psychological).
8. To understand the concept of self-esteem; its relation to performance and success; and the sources, institutions, and images that affect self-esteem (educational and psychological).

A child who is in the second stage, the transitional phase, realizes his or her lack of absolute acceptance by the white world. The individual withdraws from the dominant culture and tries to identify with his or her culture of origin, immersing himself or herself in the values and lifestyle of that culture. This is when many West Indian adolescents begin to wear dreadlocks, to rebel against their parents' Eurocentric view, and to talk emotionally of "Mother Africa." In other words, they do not necessarily have a true understanding and a true appreciation of their history; rather, their reaction reflects a loss of culture, feelings of rejection, and a need to grasp anything left of their cultural pride. This is the most difficult stage for both parents and children. They all have to acknowledge racism and discrimination. The main affect is one of frustration and anger, and behavior is generally militant. A youth's interpersonal relations tend to become limited mainly to his or her own cultural group. Therapy has to be both extensive and intensive, tapping many modalities (affective, interpersonal, educational, behavioral, cognitive, structural) and many systems (individual, family, extended family, church, and community).

A child or adolescent who is in the final, or transcendent, stage of acculturation may not need psychological therapy as such (at least not for acculturation matters), because he or she has become bicultural and uses the experiences from both cultural groups to best fit his or her own circumstances.

As can be seen from this discussion, Bowen's systems therapy, which views therapy as a self-change process and which portrays the therapist as a teacher (as described in Chapter 13), is quite compatible with the needs of West Indian families.

PHASE III. PSYCHOLOGICAL TREATMENT PROCESS

The greater the cultural differences between therapist and client, the greater the challenge to maintain the therapeutic relationship. These cultural differences can dominate the relationship and affect therapeutic progress. With an immigrant family, the therapist's efforts to "cross over" may have to be greater than for a family with values and customs similar to the therapist's. I have found that a combination of Lazarus's broad-based, multimodal approach, Minuchin's structural approach, and Bowen's family dynamics approach is the most helpful in addressing the psychological problems faced by West Indian families and in easing the "joining" or "crossing-over" process. As has been demonstrated above, the initial stages of therapy with immigrant families tend to be very educational, unless there is a crisis because of some traumatic incident. However, once the individual or family is familiar with the various systems, and if the problem persists (at times therapy with immigrant families may be merely educational), then a more psychological approach to treatment is needed.

Applying Multimodal Therapy with West Indians

Multimodal assessment, with its multilayered approach, focuses on behaviors that are impeding the happiness and acculturation of immigrant families. The therapist will observe and ask what makes an individual sad, frightened, angry, anxious, timid, and so forth. He or she will also observe what type of behaviors the individual displays when feeling these emotions: Is the individual avoiding, violent, and so forth? Generally, when maladaptive behaviors are present, behavior therapy will be implemented. Thus clients will be taught to practice prescribed exercises, whether these take the form of relaxation, meditation, assertiveness training, or modeling. Behavioral contracts will be set up, whereby the client is rewarded for compliance and deprived of privileges for noncompliance. The works of behaviorists such as Skinner (1974), Bandura (1969), Wolpe (1969), Meichenbaum (1977), and Jacobson (1938) can all be applied, depending on the nature of the problem. As mentioned above, it is highly common in multimodal therapy to begin intervening in the first interview to alleviate stress, rather than waiting until the full assessment procedure is completed. For example, if a child says he or she is stuttering because of feeling very nervous, Jacobson's progressive relaxation can be applied in the first session. In a sense, this will seem like a "gift" to the family, because a direct relationship between therapy and alleviation of problems has been demonstrated. The therapist's credibility has been established as well.

There is a strong correlation among one's cognition, affect, and behaviors. How one feels (affect) determines to a large extent how one behaves or thinks. Likewise, how one thinks influences how one feels or behaves. As a result, while I agree with Brice (1982) that West Indians "have a covert agreement among themselves not to reveal feelings" (p. 131), I do not agree that "the therapist's efforts to amplify feelings could be threatening" (p. 131), and that therefore "questions aimed at feelings will reach a dead end" (p. 131). In my experience with West Indian families, including the men, I have seen a profound need to express feelings once the therapist has established credibility. The stoicism and apparent coldness are learned behaviors, but with the change of roles for men (even in the West Indies), a more nurturing side is striving to emerge. I recommend addressing the affective side by exploring feelings in an empathetic manner. Domokos-Cheng Ham (1989a, 1989b) discusses how the therapist can "join" with immigrant families in an empathetic manner. Essentially, this author talks about the interactive process, the dyadic relationship between therapist and client, and the therapist's ability to convey emotional sensitivity. Gladstein (1983), Rogers (1975b), and Asby (1975) have all emphasized the value of the therapist's listening for feelings.

As researchers and academicians, we have a tendency to look for specificity. Thus, when we encounter imprecise quantities such as feelings and empathy, we attempt to dismiss them because these abstract constructs cannot be measured. I believe that teaching a client to express affect is a process. Although it is important to proceed cautiously in any attempt to uncover unconscious feelings, there is no doubt that West Indians, when faced with their children's maladaptive behaviors, express some feelings very openly. It is expressed in ways such as this: "I don't understand. This is not the way we behave. I feel frustrated. I am sending my child back home." What they are saying is that they cannot cope. Threatening to send children back to the West Indies (after waiting so long to be reunited with them) is the ultimate expression of pain, fear, and anger. Therapy must address these feelings, as well as teach the parents coping skills. The important factor to note here is that while the therapist may be affectively empathetic, he or she must also maintain "cognitive empathetic skills in perceiving, categorizing and making sense" of the client's feelings (Domokos-Cheng Ham, 1989a, p. 38). The idea, then, is not merely to feel what the client is feeling, but to comprehend and act on what the client is feeling. In my experience with West Indian families, affective therapy is best introduced somewhere between the middle and the end of the therapeutic process. However, if the need arises earlier, the therapist should assist the client in amplifying his or her feelings.

Exploring how thoughts influence emotions and behavior, the therapist may try to examine the client's belief (cognition) systems. Examining the client's belief that his or her child "should, ought to, must" do well may help shed some light on the undue pressure that West Indian parents sometimes place on their children, albeit unintentionally. Albert Ellis's (1974) rational–emotive therapy (RET), which is a cognitive, behavioral, and affective approach to treatment, is quite relevant to immigrant families for the following reasons:

1. RET does not require the client to give up his or her values and cultural reality; therefore, the client does not have to endorse the therapist's culture in order to get well. RET is a value-free form of therapy because it helps the client to achieve his or her goals within his or her own sociocultural context. Problems usually arise when the client's new belief system is in conflict with his or her cultural belief system. Thus a client who no longer shares the views of his or her traditional culture may experience cognitive dissonance, which has to be worked through. In such a case, the client can be taught that it is not so "awful" if his or her goals or values have to be changed in order

to function in this society. Similarly, the client can be taught that maintaining his or her traditional values is also acceptable.
2. RET is proactive, short-term, and goal-directed.
3. It provides the client with a link among his or her thoughts, affect, and behavior.
4. Rational beliefs are logical. Therefore, when a male client believes, for instance, that coming to the United States has destroyed his manhood, he is made to recognize through RET that manhood is not so fragile a concept that any event can destroy it.

The important thing to keep in mind is that with this cognitive approach to therapy, many of a client's irrational thoughts can be examined. Therefore, parents who simply expect their children to like the cultural change merely because they did, or to do well because the opportunity is here, or to acculturate with minimal difficulty can benefit from Ellis's RET.

Interpersonal relations is the area in which immigrant children experience the most difficulty in school. McNicol (1991) has outlined, from the children's perspective, several areas of adjustment that children go through when they are reunited with their families. Many children fall at each end of the continuum—unassertiveness leading to withdrawal, or aggression leading to violence or disruptive behavior. Teaching alternative ways of coping with problem situations via role play, assertiveness training, and social skills training should aid in addressing this problem. In addition, teaching children to cope with peer taunts and to understand the sociocultural differences between their native countries and the United States are some ways in improving their interpersonal relationships.

In order to improve poor self-esteem (a problem commonly seen in immigrant children), it can be helpful to explore how they perceive themselves with questions such as "What do you dislike or like about yourself?", and then to observe how these images influence moods, sensations, and behaviors. A child may complain persistently about unpleasant sensations, such as aches and pains. Often this is the child's way of communicating stress in dealing with the cultural transition. Cognitive–behavioral therapy will address the child's anxieties, but parents also have to be taught how not to reinforce or cultivate the anxiety by allowing the child to skip school. Whenever West Indian parents come into conflict with the school system, an option they tend to consider is keeping the child out of school for a few days, hoping that the problem will have simply disappeared by the time the child returns.

Many of them are unaware of terms—and realities—such as "educational neglect," and these must be taught to them.

What can be seen in examining the multimodal approach is that when therapy is dealing with behavior, affect, sensation, imagery, cognition, and interpersonal factors, the emphasis is essentially educational. The therapist offers guidance, displays caring, modifies faulty styles, corrects misconceptions, provides information, and delivers the support necessary for the client to attain his or her goals. In selecting which problems and which modality to address first, Lazarus (1976) recommends starting with the most obvious problem and using the most logical procedure. This will overcome the penchant for making straightforward problems needlessly complicated.

A Systems (Educational) Approach

Bowen's (1978) systems approach emphasizes the importance of communicating strategically within the family context. His concept of the "coach" is very applicable in working with West Indian families. Rather than meeting with the family, Bowen has the person who came to therapy coach other family members into emotionally mature relationships with one another. I have found this concept very helpful, because it is so difficult to get an entire West Indian family to come in to therapy. Since the men are so resistant and tend to deny the therapist adequate entry, using a coach may be the next most effective approach. In addition, the term "family therapy" can be quite threatening to West Indians, who may surmise that the entire family is being seen as dysfunctional. Bowen's coaching, which makes it unnecessary for the entire family to be present simultaneously, is further useful because West Indian parents often have difficulty engaging in discussions in the presence of their children, which is the typical mode of family therapy. Still another advantage of this technique is that members who may not have otherwise become involved in therapy may be treated. I have found that the best coach is the eldest male child. Although the mother is traditionally the intermediary between the father and the children, in the final analysis she is expected to side with the father, especially in the presence of the children. The eldest son, by virtue of being a male and an elder offspring, is the one who can most readily gain the respect of the younger siblings; he can also get the attention of his parents, especially his father, because of his seniority in the hierarchical family structure.

Bowen's interview technique of instructing family members to attend to one another and distinguish between thoughts and feelings is helpful in fostering more constructive contact between father and son or mother and daughter. His emphasis on person-to-person relationships (the relationships the family members have with one another) is helpful in counteracting the vulnerability that individual members feel when the entire family is against one family member. Moreover, Bowen's technique of tracing multigenerational family emotional patterns helps to differentiate the individual, since he or she can confront the family's arbitrary rules with a defined sense of self.

In addition, I have found Bowen's emphasis on personal responsibility and respect for individual boundaries very appealing to West Indian adolescents. Many adolescents who are attempting to distance themselves from their families through individuation and differentiation welcome this shifting of the family process to their own individuality. However, the therapist ought to be mindful of the deeply rooted importance of the family for West Indians. Using the approach of creating distance from family may make the individual at a later point feel shallow, in spite of his or her attempts at independence. It is best to encourage members to negotiate their individuation within the family. I have found that individuals much more readily embrace a feeling of reconnection to their families that allows some level of independence. Therefore distancing, as discussed by Bowen, should not take the form of complete differentiation from family for West Indians; rather, it should emphasize maintaining family contacts, while advocating emotional expressiveness with the families. The therapist has to teach the individual client to be prepared at each stage of differentiation to deal with the family's reactions, which may be feelings of rejection and betrayal. It should be noted that the Bowenian systems model does fit West Indian families in that it emphasizes self-determination, a concept very much endorsed in West Indian society.

A Structural Approach

Minuchin's (1974) structural family therapy approach, which emphasizes hierarchies within the family, is very relevant to West Indian culture. Parents and grandparents are usually in favor of Minuchin's emphasis on generational boundaries, instead of approaches that emphasize equal rights for all family members. By actively restructuring the family interactions, rather than relying on expressions of feelings to create change, the therapist helps to realign the family's boundaries. This approach is particularly helpful in aiding in the process of acculturation, since Minuchin emphasizes that the individual's symptoms can be traced to the family's failure to accommodate its structure to the changing environmental requirements. Like many other first-generation immigrants, West Indians often have difficulty "letting go" and endorsing the concept of biculturalism. Minuchin's approach helps the parents recognize that the children need to become involved in American society in order to assimilate with minimal difficulty. Therefore, when therapy challenges the family structure, the family is moved to examine the enmeshment syndrome (so typical in West Indian families) that may be impeding cultural adjustment. In addition, Minuchin's use of the extended family as an integral component of therapy is very effective with West Indians, since the extended family plays a pivotal role in West Indian family life.

PHASE IV. EMPOWERMENT TREATMENT PROCESS

The final stage of the treatment process is the empowering of the family via a multisystems approach. Boyd-Franklin (1989) examines the importance of intervening at various levels—individual, family, extended family, church, community, and social services. There is little doubt that this approach can be quite effective, because it provides a flexible set of guidelines for intervention with West Indian immigrants. This approach also recognizes that within the West Indian community, the idea that "it takes a whole community to raise a child" is fully endorsed by most people. Immigrant families are generally not aware of some systems (educational, legal, community), and empowering them to use all of the support systems available to them is cricial to the acculturation process. The use of these systems can be implemented at any stage in therapy, but the families *must* be aware of all potential systems before therapy is terminated so that they can tap into them readily if the need arises. Encouraging individuals to embrace the support of their extended family and of people who are not blood relatives in areas such as child care and education may help in preventing personal difficulties.

The use of the church in therapy with West Indians is also very relevant, because of the important role religion plays in the life of West Indian families. The church can serve as a valuable social service in times of crisis, particularly for single parents. West Indian elders have also used churches as points of socialization and sources of help with providing child care. The therapist should suggest the church as a support system, and may even seek permission from the family to talk to the priest or minister, in order to ascertain what role the church can play in the therapeutic process.

Of course, it is also important for the therapist to recognize the significant influence of folk beliefs in West Indian religious society. Leininger (1973) has recommended using both indigenous practitioners' skills and professional practices. I do not believe it is necessary for a therapist to conduct spiritual counseling or to even have a referral list for practitioners of obeah, since the therapist has to be knowledgeable to venture into this form of treatment and comfortable with this procedure to make such a referral. However, it is necessary for the therapist to understand that opposition to the family's seeking the help of such practitioners may impede the psychotherapeutic process. I have always provided emotional support to my clients who felt they were victims of bewitchment, and have asked them to keep me abreast of what happened after their visits to the spiritists.

The therapist must also help the family find out what after-school programs exist in their communities, since allegations of neglect are sometimes brought against working West Indian parents whose young children are at home alone after school. The families need to be taught that this is frowned upon in American society and that child care programs can be used. Boyd-Franklin (1989) has recommended that therapists should keep a file on these different services so that they can mobilize them when necessary. This kind of tapping of available resources is sometimes the most important interaction in facilitating the possibility of treatment.

In addition, the therapist needs to be knowledgeable about the legal system as it applies to immigration policies and to be familiar with at least one immigration attorney, because of the illegal immigration status of many West Indian families. (The Center for Immigrant Rights [see Appendix VI] can provide the names of attorneys from West Indian backgrounds.) Knowing about the immigration laws is important, both in order to be sensitive to families' fears regarding their immigrant status and to be able to help them with specific information—for example, that children cannot be denied a public education because of their immigrant status (a fact of which most West Indian families are unaware).

In using the Multi-CMS approach to treat West Indian families, a therapist can explore a broad spectrum of techniques to address the needs of this population. The following case example shows how this comprehensive approach can be practically implemented.

A CASE EXAMPLE

The following case example is a practical illustration of the Multi-CMS approach to therapy with West Indian families.

The Matthews family was referred for therapy by the school psychologist because of the academic and behavioral problems of their two sons, Michael and Kendall, ages 7 and 9, respectively. The eldest child, Taiesha, age 13, was also having academic difficulties; she was failing all courses except gym. Mr. Matthews was originally from Jamaica, and Mrs. Matthews from Trinidad and Tobago. They had met in Jamaica, where Mrs. Matthews spent two years after completing high school in Trinidad. They had been married for 14 years, although eight years after they married Mrs. Matthews migrated to the United States "for a better life and to give my children the chance to get a good education." The children lived in Jamaica with their father and paternal grandparents. Michael was 1 year old when his mother left home, Kendall was 3, and Taiesha was 7. Since Mrs. Matthews had come to the United States on a holiday visa, but had decided to stay on doing domestic work, she had lived for three years illegally in this country. In that time, she was unable to visit her children in Jamaica because she would not have been allowed re-entry into the United States. She was later sponsored by her employer and obtained permanent residency (approximately five years after leaving home). She immediately sponsored the other members of her family, who were now here. Although they were not legal permanent residents yet, she expected them to become so within the next few months. When the family joined Mrs. Matthews, the children were then 6, 8, and 12. Currently the household was comprised of the nuclear family, a maternal aunt and uncle, and the maternal grandmother. The children had not seen the paternal grandparents with whom they lived in Jamaica since they left the island.

These background data were sent by the school psychologist along with the referring information. In addition, there were allegations of possible child abuse and educational neglect because of the children's excessive absences from school. School officials were strongly considering placing both boys in special education because of their emotional disturbances, and Taiesha in special education because of a learning disability. However, they agreed to withhold special educa-tion placement until psychotherapeutic intervention occurred.

Initial Session

As had been agreed on the telephone, all members of the nuclear family came in for the first session. The therapist, after greeting the family, began the treatment process by asking the parents to discuss the problem as they understood it. Mrs. Matthews looked frustrated because Mr. Matthews was very angry that the family "had to be seen as crazy and abusive." He sat away from the rest of the family and did not say anything for the first 15 minutes. Mrs. Matthews explained much of what was mentioned in the referral, and the children were generally quiet. The therapist (who was a young, female clinical psychologist) at first found it necessary to address some of the family's misconceptions about the range of clients who seek counseling. The therapist also agreed with Mr. Matthews that many families are labeled abusive when in fact they are using culturally sanctioned ways of disciplining their children. At this juncture, Mr. Matthews "joined" with the therapist by sharing his frustration with this system. By conceptualizing the problem in a manner consistent with the family's cultural experiences and beliefs, the therapist gained credibility with Mr. Matthews. The therapist also used this session to enlighten the family about some basic social and cultural differences, such as sleeping arrangements, educational neglect, and the meaning of child abuse in American society. Sensitivity to the children's presence was taken into consideration, since the therapist wanted to respect the hierarchical family structure and not reveal too much in the presence of the children. Both Mr. and Mrs. Matthews said at the end of the session how much they had learned about educational, social, and cultural differences. The therapist had given to the family a "gift," and the family already saw the therapist as "credible" after the first session. The therapeutic process was explained, and the family agreed to give therapy a chance for at least one month.

Gathering Information; Outlining Goals; Empowerment

Both the first and the second sessions were spent gathering information, as well as engaging in the treatment process. The WICAB (Appendix II) was used as a guide. The second session was quite enlightening, since several issues were revealed as problems within the family:

1. Mr. Matthews's unemployment.
2. The children's feeling that they did not belong in the school and that their parents did not understand them.
3. Taiesha's embarrassment about her parents' accent and cultural values.
4. The maternal grandmother's attitude toward her son-in-law because her daughter was now the breadwinner (working two jobs).
5. The spanking of all the children by extended family members.
6. The parents' belief that Taiesha "had gotten rude."
7. The endorsement of the folk belief that "it is possible someone in Jamaica envied us because they heard we were doing well and put something on the children."

8. The fear that the children "will be deported home if they continue to give trouble in school."

The therapist continued to engage in the treatment process by explaining the educational and legal rights of the family. At the end of the session, the family was also given homework—reading two handbooks for immigrants (one on the educational and social systems and one on special education). At the end of this session, some goals were outlined; these included empowering the family to use the educational support systems in their communities in order to help the children in math and reading. The therapist also supported the family's decision to visit a spiritist by asking to be kept abreast of the results of their meetings with the obeah practitioner. In the meantime (between sessions), the therapist sent a letter to the school explaining to the principal that supplemental instruction in the English language (SIEL) might prove to be beneficial for all of the children. Goals also involved teaching all adults in the household alternative ways of disciplining children, as well as examining the effect of family role change on the family's stability.

Empowerment through Extended Family; Implementation of the Educational and Psychological Treatment Processes

There was much resistance from members of the extended family to coming in for treatment, because they did not think that the problems with the children were caused by them. So the therapist suggested making a home visit, and the third session of family therapy was conducted at home. As agreed, the entire family was present upon the therapist's arrival. The family was more responsive to therapy's being conducted in the home. In addressing the resistance, the therapist did not agree or disagree with the extended family's attitude that they did not need therapy, but rather spoke of contributions family members could make in helping to solve the problem. Resistance was diminished considerably as each family member explored ways in which he or she could be of more assistance. The aunt and uncle agreed to help in the areas of remediation and in spending more time with the children. This session also focused briefly on what constitutes child abuse. Extended family members recognized that they had been unaware of the legal ramifications of engaging in corporal punishment. Subsequent sessions with the adults were also educational in nature, in that the focus was on the emotional stress that children experience as a result of migration and their concomitant shift in value orientation. The differences in the school structure and expectations, test-taking styles, and so forth were all examined.

By this time the family had agreed to continue with therapy for another month, and the extended family members had agreed to come in to the clinic. At this juncture both family and group therapy were being provided on a weekly basis. From the fourth session up to the end of therapy, Michael and Kendall joined a group for young boys, while Taiesha joined a group for teenage girls. In both groups, issues such as coping with peer pressure, social skills and assertiveness training (to assist with interpersonal relations), building self-esteem, understanding the educational differences in test-taking styles, and coping with their fears about acculturation were addressed. In addition, Michael and Kendall were taught self-control separately from the group, while Taiesha's embarrassment about her parents' accent and her father's refusal to treat her as a teenager were discussed in a family session.

Family therapy was held with the adults only, to address the conflict as a result of family role changes. The children were asked to sit outside when marital issues were being discussed. Mr. and Mrs. Matthews both felt that having the children sit in on the therapy session would result in their knowing too much about marital conflicts. This wish was respected, but Mrs. Matthews's mother, who was also a catalyst in creating stress on Mr. Matthews, was expected to be in attendance. RET explored their cultural beliefs about men being the sole breadwinners. In addition, the role conflict for children and parents was addressed in family therapy by helping family members to establish some individuation, but at the same time maintaining family cohesiveness. Group therapy for Taiesha also addressed how adolescents can prepare their families at each stage of the differentiation process. Furthermore, group therapy focused on helping Taiesha to understand her parents' perception of the hierarchies within the family and what it meant in relation to respect.

In addition, the family members were taught the principles of behaviorism and ways in which they might have directly or indirectly reinforced negative behaviors in one another. A behavior modification program was set up at home, whereby the children were reinforced for good behavior and effort in school. After obtaining the parents' informed consent, the teachers were sent letters explaining what was being done and how it would be helpful for them to send home a daily behavior checklist so that the family could appropriately reward the children. The children were then further rewarded by the therapist during group therapy time.

It was not until about the sixth family session that feelings pertaining to the children's not feeling loved by their parents were addressed. The children's feelings about their father's "abuses" and their mother's extended hours at work were also discussed. Kendall was particularly emotional as he talked about not feeling loved because his father never hugged him. This session focused on touching as a form of communicating, and everyone was asked to hug the person nearest him or her. Then all were told to hug whichever family members they so desired. Interestingly, no one reached to hug Mr. Matthews until this was pointed out by the therapist. At that point, he said he would like to hug everyone and proceeded to do so. From that session onward, homework involved daily tactile forms of communication. In the meantime, the reality that Mrs. Matthews needed to work in order to pay the bills was explored, but all family members decided they would assist in domestic matters so that she would be free to engage in family activities once she got home. Mr. Matthews, who had refused to cook before, agreed to do so, so that Mrs. Matthews would not have to get up early to cook before leaving for work. In addition, Mr. Matthews agreed to enroll in an educational program to obtain his high school diploma while still seeking employment.

The ninth session in treatment was educational again, with family members encouraged to establish contact with more social support systems. Taiesha joined a youth group that was monitored by West Indian adults in the community. She built a wonderful network of friends who had themselves gone through cultural conflicts while in transition. Mr. Matthews eventually agreed to join a black male self-esteem group, which focused on such issues as "the invisibility syndrome" as it pertains to black males and the psychology of being a black male in this society. All family members agreed to become members of their local church. The therapist established contact with the pastor, who introduced the family to the congregation at Mass.

In the meantime, the children continued to show academic delays, but behavior problems had decreased considerably. The therapist visited the school with the parents and suggested at a school-based support team meeting what representatives of each discipline (psychologist, nurse, social worker, teachers) could be responsible for in assisting these children. Although this was a difficult task, given the bureaucracy in the education system, they did agree to refrain from placing the children in special education for at least two years.

The success of this case may have been a result of the holistic approach to therapy. The Multi-CMS approach, while demanding, covered all areas that caused distress within the family unit. In addition, the concept that "it takes a whole community to raise a child" certainly aided the members of this family in arming and empowering themselves as they attempted to acculturate to American society.

PART III

IMPLICATIONS

Training Implications for Mental Health Workers, Teachers, Speech Evaluators, and Parents

The ultimate goal of multicultural education and cross-cultural psychology is to increase the excellence of all teachers and counselors, regardless of their students' or clients' cultural background. In my experience with graduate students, I have found that while they are able to recognize the limitations in their training, they simply do not have the skills to address the needs of the culturally different. Therefore, much of my supervision involves emphasizing what appropriate approaches *can* work, rather than just pointing out what will not work.

EXAMINING PERSONAL VALUES:
A PREREQUISITE FOR INTERVENTION

Many therapists and other professionals are unaware of their own biases and subjectivity, and bringing their own values and their impact on treatment to awareness is a prerequisite for working with culturally different clients. By looking at their own cultural upbringing; by examining their feelings, attitudes, and behaviors toward people of different cultures; and by being exposed to several culturally different people—the interaction approach (Triandis & Brislin, 1984)—clinicians and other professionals can become more alert to the cultural relativity of their values. I have found with my trainees that sometimes merely discussing cultural differences creates much pain, especially for nonwhite trainees, who feel that their culture was never considered in theory development. White trainees express their resentment at being labeled discriminatory and prejudiced. Therefore, initially, trainees experience much difficulty with this process and even prefer not to deal with it at all.

I do a fundamental exercise with all my trainees. First, they are asked to identify their ethnic and cultural background, and what they like and dislike about their own ethnic and cultural group. They are also asked to think about (not necessarily to say in the presence of others) what they dislike about other ethnic and cultural groups. Next, they are presented with facts about other groups or cultures through reading materials and lectures. (See Table 15.1 for a breakdown on basic West Indian cultural values that differ from American ones.) Finally, on an ongoing basis, they are expected to attend cross-cultural continuing education seminars—a sort of weekly or monthly roundtable.

It is vitally important that the training atmosphere be sensitive to the trainees' fears. Moreover, trainees must come to recognize a direct correlation between this exercise and their effectiveness as culturally sensitive therapists.

The remainder of this chapter will focus on training implications for school psychologists, other mental health workers, teachers, and speech/language evaluators, as well as the role of mental health workers in the training of West Indian parents.

TRAINING IMPLICATIONS FOR MENTAL HEALTH WORKERS

Training Implications for School Psychologists

Chapter 11 has illustrated the biases in various WISC-R subtests with respect to West Indians. In spite of these biases, the WISC-R is still used to label children as "retarded" and as a primary tool in determining special education placement. To be more accurate in their assessment of intelligence, school psychologists can use the Digit Span subtest in tabulating the verbal IQ, instead of or in addition to the General Information subtest (the most culturally biased subtest). By

Table 15.1. A Selected Comparison of West Indian and American Cultural Values

West Indian	American
Family rights are most important.	Individual rights are most important.
Teachers are as respected as parents.	Teachers are not automatically respected.
Children do not have much independence and are expected to obey and respect their elders.	Children have much independence.
Family relations are very close.	Family relations are not always close.
Siblings sleep with one another in the same bedroom and in some cases in the same bed, even if they are of different genders.	Only children of the same gender sleep in the same bedroom.
West Indians do not look steadily at a respected person's eyes.	American maintain eye contact in most situations.
West Indians, while they think of the future, tend to be oriented to the present.	Americans constantly plan for the future—for example, their retirement.
Mental illness is seen in a spiritual sense.	Mental illness is seen in a more philosophical sense.

using this test, school officials should be able to obtain a better idea of a child's potential.

It is important in assessing children to gain an understanding of their current performance as well as their potential ability. In writing psychological reports, I tend to examine children's strengths and to note how these strengths can be used to maximize their potential and/or overcome their weaknesses. In other words, instead of merely reporting scores, psychological reports ought to be more descriptive. Furthermore, it may prove to be quite beneficial if children are allowed to go beyond their ceiling points in the nonverbal subtests to see whether they do in fact master the manipulation of blocks and puzzles (see Chapter 11). Here again, the report can provide two scores—one reflecting the child's actual performance, and the other the child's potential given his or her strengths. Armour-Thomas (in press) has found that when teachers capitalize on the strengths in higher-order thinking that low-achieving students bring to academic tasks, then not only do such students become more rigorous in their thinking, but they acquire new knowledge and extend their existing knowledge more readily.

A colleague and I (Gopaul-McNicol & Shapiro, 1992) have discussed the learning styles of children and described how school psychologists can assist teachers in bringing the diverse cultural learning styles of children into the classroom. As noted in earlier chapters, in the West Indies the approach to teaching is auditorily mediated, since a typical classroom has few or no visual aids. It is therefore not surprising that West Indian children's highest WISC-R subtest score tends to be on Digit Span, which taps auditory short-term memory. I have found (Gopaul-McNicol, 1990) that West Indian children score higher than white American students on this subtest.

Moreover, the question of learning disability versus mental retardation versus educational deprivation (discussed in Chapter 11) must be considered in working with West Indian children. In conducting an assessment of West Indian children, I always do a differential assessment of mental retardation from educational deprivation (see Chapter 11).

The purpose of testing is to see how children are functioning intellectually, how much they learned in their countries of origin, what their strengths and weaknesses are relative to American culture and to their native cultures, and whether they have the ability or the potential to learn and assimilate into this new culture. Although the WISC-R may not adequately sample West Indian students' prior learning experiences, it can help in assessing what children know relative to American culture and to what extent they have acquired the skills relevant to academic success in the American school system. The WISC-R is also helpful in assessing how quickly children can learn under optimal conditions. Therefore I do not recommend throwing this assessment tool out, but rather being aware of the ethical responsibilities associated with multicultural assessment.

A psychologist assessing someone from a culturally different background must be aware that there is some potential for unintentional bias and unreliability, because it is so difficult to shed one's own ethnocentrism. Most importantly, school psychologists ought to be familiar with the argument against the "culturally deficient" model. As Samuda (1975) has stated, "Minorities should be viewed no longer as culturally deficient or culturally disadvantaged, but culturally different" (p. 9). I also endorse Baratz and Baratz's (1970) statement that "education should take as its primary goal to produce a bi-cultural child who is capable of functioning both in his subculture and in the mainstream" (p. 43).

Language plays a vital role in assessment of children, as Chapter 11 has noted. In the West Indies, while children are taught to read and write standard English in the classroom, they speak West Indian Creole at home. Thus many words can be misinterpreted in testing. One would not want these children's education to be based on their below-average performance on an IQ test, such as the WISC-R (see the section below on training implications for speech/language evaluators).

The classroom climate is of major importance in learning. Often immigrant children say that they do not like the school or classroom, because they are teased by their peers about their accent or foods they bring for lunch. School psychologists can offer advice to teachers about social activities that can be conducted in the classroom. Pasternak (1986) has suggested many cultural activities that teachers can use in the classroom to increase cultural sensitivity. In addition, school psychologists must involve students in classroom training to increase multicultural awareness, enhance intergroup communications, and build the self-esteem of all students. Furthermore, school psychologists can prepare school personnel on how to cope with West Indian children who may be experiencing culture shock or post-traumatic stress disorder (see Chapters 11 and 12).

Training Implications for All Mental Health Workers

In addition to everything else that has been presented in this book, especially in Part II, it is important that mental health workers be willing to use people in the community as paraprofessionals, so that they can bridge the gap between the institution and their clients' world. This will enable therapists to learn about and understand the community firsthand from individuals who respect the people residing there. Elliston (1985) and my colleagues and I (Gopaul-McNicol et al., 1991) also recommend teaching newly arrived immigrants the basic educational and social differences between the West Indies and the United States.

In addition, literature to dispel myths about West Indians should be disseminated to workers. The main myths are the following:

1. West Indians arriving in the United States are only interested in making money; therefore, they work several jobs at the expense of their families.

2. West Indian men are abusive to their women because they are so controlling.
3. A patriarchal structure is universal in West Indian families.
4. West Indians do not want to become U.S. citizens.
5. Black West Indians think they are superior to other blacks.
6. Black West Indians do not consider themselves black at all.
7. West Indians do not believe in mental illness.

Many clinicians do not know that in many less developed countries, such as the West Indies, psychiatric hospitals are structurally and functionally different from those in more developed countries, such as the United States. Fewer people are hospitalized, and when they are, it is because a disturbance is chronic and/or conspicuous. Thus first-generation West Indians see hospitals as a last resort; they are influenced by memories of relatives and friends in their homelands who never returned from the hospitals. In the West Indies, most people who are mentally disturbed are treated as outpatients for several years before they enter hospitals (if they ever do). In addition to their general attitude about mental illness (see Chapters 11 and 12), West Indians have never been exposed to the type of resources or services that exist in this country (probably because of economic reasons and lack of professionals). Therefore, it is only when a disorder is severe that they come in for treatment.

An opportunity for trainees or clinicians to role-play West Indian patients should also be included in this training program. Boyd-Franklin (1989) has recommended enacting scenarios of families that staff or trainees are actually treating. This generates much clinical insight into the West Indian culture, especially when the trainees share their conflicts and stereotypes. When the trainees are experiencing difficulty, the supervisor can intervene by assuming the role of a family member and demonstrating to the trainees the correct responses. This can be very helpful in helping trainees to see how a family may be responding to them.

Understanding psychopathology across cultures should be a major part of clinical training. Chapter 11 explores how West Indians may be misdiagnosed because of their cultural spiritual beliefs and practices.

Any training program should also involve clinicians' ability to help their West Indian clients address the issue of racism. Many West Indians do not know how to cope with racism, since in the West Indies they did not experience the level of institutionalized racism that exists in the United States.

In recent years there has been much debate about the use of role models in therapy. DeFour (1991) found that "same race role models and mentors appear to be better facilitators of minority students' career development and retention" (p. 1). In my clinical work with West Indian families (especially male children), I include role models of the same race and, if possible, the same culture as part of the therapeutic process. Every other session for five minutes, I have a guest speaker come in to talk about his or her achievement and describe how he or she was able to overcome various obstacles, from peer pressure to racism.

Another technique that I find quite beneficial and useful in working with West Indian families is videotaping—a technique used by many family therapists, such as Boyd-Franklin (1989). By showing the videotape of a session, the therapist is better able to point out to the family their dysfunctional communication patterns; moreover, after seeing themselves, many individuals come to a better understanding of how they are perceived by others. It encourages much interaction and even results in laughter and the breakdown of familial tensions.

Chapters 12 and 14 have described the importance of home visits; this cannot be emphasized enough in working with West Indian families. This technique is particularly helpful in getting the men (who are the most resistant) in for therapy and in creating therapist credibility. Many West Indians feel honored that a therapist is interested enough in them to make a home visit. They then feel "obligated" to come in for therapy. Boyd-Franklin (1989) recommends a "buddy system" for therapists who feel uncomfortable visiting homes in dangerous neighborhoods.

In working with West Indian families, as with most immigrants, the concept of the multidisciplinary team is very important. Teachers, doctors, and nurses, in addition to social workers, psychologists, and psychiatrists, are vital team members in doing psychotherapy with West Indian families. Traditionally, West Indians respond more readily to the educational and medical institutions because of the tremendous respect teachers, doctors, and nurses are given in the West Indies. Thus the presence of a teacher (particularly in the case of children) and a nurse or doctor as part of a diagnostic team alleviates much anxiety. This also provides an introduction to some of the available support systems that the family can tap into when faced with crises.

TRAINING IMPLICATIONS FOR TEACHERS

In 1973 the American Association of Colleges for Teacher Education (AACTE) launched a forceful multicultural statement which read in part: "To endorse cultural pluralism is to understand and appreciate the differences that exist among the nation's citizens" (quoted in Dillard, 1983, p. 9). This statement clearly suggests that merely placating and accommodating racially and culturally different students are not what cultural pluralism is about. Rather, cultural pluralism requires educators to take a serious look at their curricula, which have thus far only endorsed the principle of one model American and have not yet given intrinsic respect to every individual. Current curricula treat the West Indian child as an oddity. Integrating Caribbean literature into the curricula is one way to correct this problem.

In training teachers to work with West Indian immigrant children, London (1978, 1980, 1983, 1984, 1987, 1988, 1989, 1990) has suggested that teacher training must include an understanding of the West Indian cultural background and points of cultural conflict for West Indian immigrants, in order to prevent misunderstanding in the classroom. London (1990) has further suggested that teachers should encourage immigrant children to articulate their own stories, orally or in writing. In my own experience, I have learned that teachers who integrate black and Caribbean literature into their curricula are likely to be more successful in maintaining student motivation, interest, and classroom participation. Many West Indian immigrant students mention that they feel part of the mainstream when they see themselves reflected through their culture and role models. Table 15.2 (see below) lists recommended texts that teachers can use to bring to West Indian students a part of their culture. In addition, Chapter 8 outlines the contributions of West Indians to American society in the areas of politics, entertainment, literature, science, and sports. This can be used as a source of building identity in the classroom.

Teacher Expectations

Teachers ought to be trained to understand how their unintentional biases against children from different cultures can lead to the self-fulfilling prophecy of relative academic failure among immigrant children. Short (1985) has found that if teachers believe that certain behaviors and achievements are characteristic of specific pupils, the children may internalize these perceptions over time and eventually conform to the teachers' expectations. It is therefore important to eradicate the negative stereotypes that many teachers have of West Indian students. Like counselors and other professionals, teachers have to be taught to get in touch with their biases.

Speech Patterns and Word Spellings

Teachers must be trained to understand that West Indian speech patterns are not deficient, but different. It is also important for them to know that West Indian children have as much difficulty understanding American speech patterns as the teachers have understanding West Indian speech patterns. Teachers must realize further that West Indian students will gradually exchange their British spelling and writing styles for American patterns. They should not be rushed to do so, since they are already coping with so many issues. Encouraging reading and writing will be more beneficial than constantly correcting a child. Chapter 11 discusses some of the differences in spelling, and Part 2 of Appendix II outlines some differences in the American and West Indian educational systems. The section below on speech/language evaluators is also useful for teachers.

Learning Styles

Teachers should consider the strengths and learning styles of West Indian children as remediation is offered. Dunn and Dunn (1978) and Dunn, Gemake, Jalali, and Zenhausern (1990) have emphasized that if a student fails to learn because of the way in which the teacher teaches, it is incumbent upon the teacher to change to a method that meets with greater success. This is important because current strategies are not as effective as they should be with West Indian children. This may be because instruction in the American classroom is very visual, whereas newly arrived West Indian immigrants' school experiences have been very auditory, as noted earlier. Therefore speaking rather than writing information on the board, or using audiotapes for instruction rather than visual aids (such as computers), may prove to be more successful approaches with these children.

Another difference in educational style is the type of examinations that are given. Essay tests predominate in the West Indian school system, while multiple-choice tests are more common in the United States. It takes some time for children to get used to this form of test. Some children actually feel that the teacher will not take scores on multiple-choice tests seriously, because, in their perception, essay tests truly test knowledge and multiple-choice tests are simplistic. In addition, children in the West Indies engage in a more cooperative type of learning, which fosters more dependence and sharing; in contrast, the American educational style is more independent. These differences in learning styles are critical. Teachers must both respect the West Indian style and allow sufficient time for students to adjust and adapt to the American style.

Deferring Special Education Placement

An informal assessment involving behavioral observations in several settings—classroom, playground, the home, and (if possible) the community—will help in understanding the needs, strengths, and weaknesses of a West Indian child before a referral to special education is made. Time is an important factor before determining placement. Children who were educationally deprived and are functioning two or more grades below their current placement need intensive instruction in math and reading for about three hours a day for two years before their placement is determined. The remainder of the day can be spent in the regular classroom setting. If a discrepancy still exists between achievement and intelligence or verbal and nonverbal skills after such instruction, a more restrictive setting can be considered. A program to train all school staff in understanding the experiences, learning styles, and so forth of West Indian children, and to show how best to assist in their acculturation, is strongly recommended—the children remain in their regular classes, but staff members are retrained. With the continued increase in the number of immigrant children in the United States, "pull-out" programs are increasingly less practical.

Deferring special education placement is also strongly urged when teachers suspect "emotional disturbance." Chapter 11 discusses some of the misdiagnoses that can be made by school personnel. Teachers need to be trained to understand the culture shock these students are experiencing. One black West Indian student told me it took him an entire semester to get used to being in class with so many white students. In addition, West Indians students are usually surprised at the verbal liberties afforded students and the lack of deference accorded teachers. I remember my first year at college, when, for the first time, I heard profanity used in the classroom in the presence of a professor. It was such a shock to me that I cried out. What astounded me even more was that the class continued as usual—no one else was amazed at the use of such language in the classroom. Teachers must be aware of the bewilderment and feelings of dislocation that are experienced by recently arrived immigrant students when they encounter such cultural differences in the classroom. In general, training programs are needed to educate school faculties to the language, cultural backgrounds, learning styles, and special needs of West Indian students, since these programs can forestall referrals for special education placement.

Teacher Role in Parent Training

West Indian parents often experience difficulty in understanding American education. Teachers may need to set aside time to educate parents on class programs, methodology for skill development, the purpose of study guides, homework policy, tests, the criteria for student evaluation, and what parents can do to reinforce what is being done in the school. In addition, teachers must distribute to West Indian parents information pertaining to their educational rights and responsibilities, especially if the children are being considered for special educational placement. This information is succinctly outlined in handbooks for parents (Gopaul-McNicol et al., 1991; Thomas & Gopaul-McNicol, 1991).

Recommended Texts for Inclusion in a Multicultural Curriculum

Table 15.2 presents a list of available Caribbean literature that teachers can use in their daily curriculum. These books can be obtained in the United States from Headstart Books and Crafts, 604 Flatbush Avenue, Brooklyn, New York, 11225; the telephone number is 718-469-4500 and the owner is Fritz Lewis. In England, the books can be obtained from Headstart Books and Crafts, 25 West Green Road, London N15. In Canada, they can be obtained from Third World Books and Crafts, 942 Bathurst St., Toronto, Ontario M5R 3G5; the telephone number is 416-537-8039. Teachers are encouraged to use other books that may not be on this list, if they are relevant to Caribbean culture.

TRAINING IMPLICATIONS FOR SPEECH/LANGUAGE EVALUATORS

Chapter 11 discusses the difficulty involved in linguistic assessment of West Indian children—a difficulty largely caused by the various dialects they speak. Many children are mislabeled as "speech-impaired" because their pronunciation is different, and this difference is often seen as an inferiority or deficiency because of the truncation of words ("broken English"). This can be detrimental to the West Indian child, who may then experience feelings of inferiority. Students who always thought of themselves as speaking "English" are suddenly faced with daily reminders from their teachers that, in fact, they are speaking "nonstandard" English. Such children may become so bewildered that they may socially withdraw. Several issues raised in Chapter 11 ought to be strongly considered in the training of speech/language evaluators;

Table 15.2. Caribbean Literature

Michael Anthony:	*Cricket in the Road*
	Green Days by the River
Edward Braithwaite:	*Masks*
Faustin Charles:	*Crab Track*
	The Expatriate
Zee Edgell:	*Beka Lamb*
Wilson Harris:	*Palace of the Peacock*
Roy Heath:	*A Man Come Home*
Erroll Hill:	*Three Caribbean Plays*
Merle Hodge:	*Cricket Crack Monkey*
Louis James:	*The Islands in Between*
Errol John:	*Moon on a Rainbow Shawl*
George Lamming:	*In the Castle of My Skin*
Earl Lovelace:	*The School Master*
	The Dragon Can't Dance
V. S Naipaul:	*A House for Mr. Biswas*
V. S. Reid:	*New Day*
Samuel Selvon:	*Ways of Sunlight*
Derek Walcott:	*Dream on Monkey Mountain*
Dennis Williams:	*Other Leopards*

The following handbooks provide helpful practical information for West Indian immigrants:

S. Gopaul-McNicol, T. Thomas, & G. Irish: *A Handbook for Immigrants: Some Basic Educational and Social Issues in the United States of America.*

T. Thomas & S. Gopaul-McNicol: *An Immigrant Handbook on Special Education in the United States of America.*

M. Pasternak: *Helping Kids Learn Multicultural Concepts: A Handbook of Strategies*

in particular, a SIEL program should be given special attention. In addition, some questions should be kept in mind by speech evaluators:

1. Is the child responding in Creole but able to understand American English? If so, then the issue involves expressive language difficulties, not receptive language delays. Expressive language delays can also be results of such emotional factors as self-esteem issues with respect to accent and pronunciation.

2. Has the child mastered social fluency (which involves body language and facial expression) but not the deep language structure (the academic language of instruction)? Social language takes

approximately two years (Elliot-Lewis, 1989), while conceptual language takes five years for total acquisition.

The main point is that speech evaluators must allow these children the time to acclimate to the American lexicon. If this time is not allowed, students may be saying one thing and teachers may be interpreting another. McNerney (1979, 1980) has identified some words that in the West Indian lexicon may have a different meaning than in Canadian or U.S. standard English. For instance, "tea" is any hot beverage, "fresh" can mean spoiled, and "hello" can be an attention-seeking device rather than a greeting. McNerney (1980) concludes that these "apparent similarities can interfere greatly with with acquisition of English as a second language" (p. 31). Valere-Meredith (1989) emphasizes that "dialect eradication is not the solution to teaching 'standard' English structures" (p. 8). Instead, like McNerney (1980), she advocates discussing the differences between "standard" English and the dialect, and then teaching the student to convert his or her own speech patterns with strategies such as tape-recorded materials and language drills. Pedagogical suggestions also include "code switching" (Edwards, 1983), which involves reinforcing the child when he or she changes his or her dialect to "standard" English.

What is apparent here is a double bind. On the one hand, children are classified as speech-impaired and are placed in special education. However, because these children speak a form of English ("broken" as it may be), it seems to obviate the necessity of speech/language training. West Indian children are frequently corrected for speaking poorly, but they receive little or no help, while their Latino and Asian peers receive extra English classes every day. Here we see the double disadvantage of West Indian children—a lowered evaluation of their linguistic abilities, but no systematic training in language remediation. It is not surprising that many children, experiencing such devaluations on a daily basis, become "hostile." Of course, if a teacher's preconceptions of a West Indian child are negative, this hostile behavior reinforces the teacher's negative stereotype of the child.

An important factor to note is that ESL methodology cannot be applied to the teaching of English to West Indian students in the same manner as it is applied to speakers of, say, Cantonese (McNerney, 1980). Spanish and Asian students are in fact learning an entirely new language. West Indian students, for the most part, already know the basic written structure of the language but need to practice the social fluency of "standard" English. Thus West Indian students are learning English as a second dialect, not as a second language. There should be no attempt to eradicate a student's dialect completely. Valere-Meredith (1983, 1985) states that to do so shows disapproval of dialects, which is likely to deter students from continuing to study and may even lead to confusion and hypercorrection. Dialect eradication has proven to be fallacious as a solution to teaching "standard" English. Craig (1966) suggests that teachers should only correct what has been taught, rather than every error the child makes. Edwards (1979) recommends a bidialectal approach, whereby a comparison is made between the West Indian dialect and "standard" English, so that students can see how the two languages are similar and how they differ. Roberts (1988) recommends meaningful distinction between "standard" English and Creole, whereby the student has exercises in pronunciation. Of course, the teacher has to have some knowledge of the West Indian dialect.

Another area to which speech evaluators need to be sensitive is the concept of illiteracy. My experiences with school personnel have led me to conclude that the concept of illiteracy in the United States is vastly different from that in the West Indies. Comments such as "The parent is illiterate, so this is why the child speaks the way he or she does" are common from teachers. Although some families from very rural areas may not have had any formal education in reading and writing, they are a minority; most West Indians will have had at least a primary school education, which does afford them minimal literacy skills. In their native countries, this is sufficient for them to manage in their small villages, but in technically advanced societies they find themselves at a disadvantage. It is important for educators to encourage such parents to enroll in adult training programs so that they can be of more assistance to their children. The training programs should focus on the acquisition of functional skills that are practical and applicable to their communities.

THE ROLE OF MENTAL HEALTH WORKERS IN PARENT TRAINING

Mental health workers can play a major role in educating immigrant parents about the educational and social differences in the U.S. system (Gopaul-McNicol et al., 1991). They can encourage them to attend PTA meetings, explain the issues of confidentiality regarding school records, help them establish contact with community resources—all in all, assist in the acculturation process. All mental health workers can teach parents alternatives to corporal punishment. Chapter 14 outlines some of the parent training programs to which mental health workers can expose parents on an ongoing basis. In summary, helping parents to understand the social and emotional adjustment difficulties their children are experiencing is of major importance in parent training.

Mental health workers also need to alert parents to the reality of special education and the need for them to question the motives of the teacher. As a rule, West Indian parents trust their children's teachers and allow placement in special education if the teachers recommend it. They need to be taught about the special education system, since this is a rather foreign concept to most of them. We (Thomas & Gopaul-McNicol, 1991) discuss this in detail. In general, assisting in the acculturation process involves nine important points:

1. Education about the differences in the education and social systems, with emphasis on alternative disciplinary strategies, the meaning of educational neglect, and the importance of attending parent–teacher meetings.
2. Family empowerment, with emphasis on their legal rights (see Chapter 14).
3. Understanding the family role changes and their effect on acculturation (see Chapter 12).
4. Improving communication between parents and children.
5. Teaching parents how to build or maintain positive self-esteem in their children.
6. Coping with racism.
7. Teaching parents what support their children need at home and the importance of prioritizing their time.
8. Teaching parents how to cope with rejection from their children because of the children's embarrassment about their parents' accent.
9. Teaching immigrants how to endorse the concept of biculturalism, so that they will not have to live between two worlds.

The question most often asked by parents is this: "How can I really raise children without disciplining them? I only know the way I was raised in the West Indies." The answer involves not only teaching parents the principles of assertive discipline, but also helping parents to recognize that since their children are the first generation of West Indian Americans, many of the traditional West Indian values will be passed on to them. Expediting the process of "Americanization" in a radical way may leave the parents feeling stripped of cultural pride. Although it is necessary for parents to understand that there are laws governing them with respect to "child abuse," they must also understand that acculturation for first-generation immigrants is a different process from acculturation for second- and third-generation immigrants. Although some of the traditional values will be passed on, inevitably their children will not have the same tremendous allegiance to West Indian culture, and the strong West Indian identity will dissipate over time as each new generation becomes more Americanized. West Indian immigrant parents ought not to be expected to abandon all of their values, because this can create much anxiety and despair, leaving them very vulnerable and immobilized in a sometimes hostile environment. West Indian parents need to be taught that the essence and beauty of their culture are some of their traditional values, and that to some extent, some of these values can be quite beneficial in helping children to cope. What immigrant families need to be taught is how to take the best from both cultures as they attempt to assimilate in their new country.

CHAPTER 16

Implications for Future Research and Clinical Work

Several issues and questions that have been raised throughout the course of this book need further investigation:

1. Further exploration of the Multi-CMS approach to treatment with West Indian families and other immigrants is needed.
2. Much more work needs to be done on diversity among West Indians. Interisland differences were not explored in detail in this book, but such diversity does exist. There needs to be discussion about the differences of people from smaller versus larger islands, as well as of French and Dutch West Indians versus British West Indians. Similarly, the differences between African West Indians and African Americans should be addressed, particularly with respect to psychotherapeutic interventions.
3. The learning styles of West Indian children need to be examined through the administration of reliable and valid instruments.
4. Folk beliefs and their impact on assessment and treatment are sensitive areas requiring further research. In like manner, biases in personality tests need to be examined.
5. A West Indian achievement test needs to be developed and standardized throughout the West Indies for use with West

Indian immigrant children upon arrival in the United States, Britain, and Canada.

6. The tendency of West Indian children to show perceptual–motor skill delays because of rotations on visual–motor tests needs to be investigated further.

7. The question of educational deprivation versus mental retardation versus learning disability ought to be explored further.

8. The effect of racism and its impact on acculturation should be investigated.

9. The effects of immigration status on the acculturation of families and educational achievement of children should be investigated.

10. Multicultural educational approaches that include the contributions of Caribbean culture are needed in all disciplines. Counselors and teachers should be required to undertake in-service training in strategies related to working with West Indian students.

11. Schools should recognize the validity of the English Creole language. The issue of ESD versus ESL instruction ought to be examined in the United States.

12. A child should be in the United States for at least two years before being placed in special education. A transitional remediation program should be implemented in the interim.

13. The effect of becoming U.S. citizens on the empowerment of West Indian families should be studied.

Appendix I

Map of the West
Indies

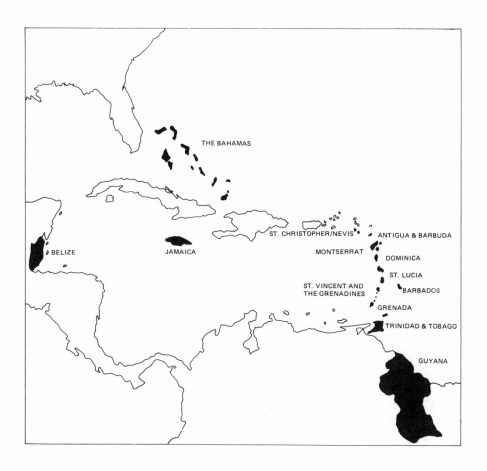

West Indian Comprehensive Assessment Battery (WICAB)

This instrument consists of two parts. Part 1 is aimed at assisting the clinician in assessing the client's various support systems; the social, emotional, and psychological functioning of the client; and the cultural transitional conflicts being experienced by the client. Part 2 provides a comparison between the education system in the West Indies and that of the United States.

PART 1: PSYCHOSOCIAL ASSESSMENT

Identifying Data

Name: Age:

Address:

Grade/class/employment:

Background Data

Were you born in this country?   Yes   No

If the client answered "no" to the question above, ask what country in the West Indies he or she was from originally.

Were you living in a rural area or an urban area?

What was your educational level prior to coming to this country? (*See Part 2 below for more detail.*)

What was your professional affiliation prior to coming to this country?

If the client answered "yes" to being born in this country, ask what country or countries his or her parents and spouse were from originally.

Country of mother: Country of father:
Country of spouse:

Were you the first person in your entire family who was born in this country?

How long have you been residing in this country?

How old were you when you came to this country?

Whom did you live with in the West Indies?

How long were you away from your parent(s) or child(ren) before reuniting with them?

How often did you see your parent(s) or child(ren while you were separated from them?

Voluntariness of Contact

Did you want to come to this country?   Yes   No

Were you expected to come because your parents moved or because of economic conditions or because you wished to receive advanced education?

Do you like it in this country?

Why/why not?

How is this country different from your home?

Family Support

Whom do you live with now?

Who is usually home when you get home from school/work?

Do you have other family members living in this country?

Where do they live?

How often do you see them?

Do you have family members living back home?

Who are they?

How often do you see/speak to/write to them?

Do they plan to come here? (*Note feelings about this separation.*)

Do you have to support any family members back home?

What is going to happen if you do not send money to them?

Do you/your parents/your spouse work?

How many hours per week do you/your parents/your spouse work?

What are some of the activities you do together?

Do you feel you are able to communicate with your parent(s)/ child(ren)/spouse?

Assess if there are role changes between men and women, parent and children, husband and wife by asking:
Who is the main breadwinner in the home?

Do you consider yourself the child of/parent to (name parents/children)? (*This is to determine if traditional familial role perceptions still exist.*)

Assess who has the power in the family.

(For Parents) Discipline

How do you discipline your children?

Do you know of alternative ways to discipline your children?

Would you be interested in learning alternative ways of disciplining your children?

Community/Social Support

Are you affiliated with any church/community organizations?
If "yes," ask:
What are they?

What is your role?
If "no," recommend this as important to aid in acculturation.

Do you have friends at school/work?

Do you have a really good friend whom you can count on if a problem arises?

Language

What language does the client speak? Standard English/West Indian Creole/other?

What language do you speak at home?

Self-Concept

(The Immigrant Self-Concept Scale [Appendix III] can also be given if this area will be the focus in treatment.)

Do you think West Indians are smart/honest/lazy?

Are you proud to say you are a West Indian?

Why/why not?

(For children) What do you want to be when you leave school?

Racial Attitude

(The Immigrant Attitude Survey [Appendix IV] can also be given to determine the client's attitudes in various other areas.)

How do you define yourself racially?

If he or she defines himself or herself as black, ask:
How do you feel about being called black?

If he or she does not define himself or herself as black, even though he or she is, explore the conflicts.

Ask the client to finish the following sentences and then discuss them in more detail:
If I had a choice, I would prefer to be white/black/other because _____

_____

I like blacks because _____

I like whites because _____

I do not like blacks because _____

I do not like whites because _____

I prefer a black/white teacher because _____

My parents view black people as _____

My parents view white people as _____

I am afraid of black people because _____

I am afraid of white people because _____

I think that black people are _____

I think that white people are _____

I think black Americans are _____

I prefer my children to have black/white friends because _____

I like being black because _____

I do not like being black because _____

Because of my skin color I cannot _____

I think I can do anything I want: Yes   No

Legal Status

(*Be aware that the family members may be circumspect. You might want to ask this at a later point. Assure them they do not have to answer.*)

Who sponsored you to come to this country?

What is your legal status?

Ask clients who are in this country illegally if they know their children's educational rights and the other rights of illegal immigrants. If they do not, inform them (see Chapter 2).

Ask clients who are in this country illegally if they know of an immigration attorney. If they do not, refer them to one or to the Center for Immigrant Rights (see Appendix VI).

Acculturation

Is this the first time you have migrated from one country to another?
If "no," ask:

Where did you migrate to prior to coming to this country?

Have there been any difficulties in readjusting to your family?
If "yes," ask the client to describe in as much detail as possible the difficulties.

Do you feel pressured to let go of your cultural values?
If "yes," ask by whom.

Do you feel pressured to maintain your cultural values or the values of your parents?

Do you feel pressured to consider yourself an African American?

What are your religious beliefs?

Stage of Acculturation

Do you feel as if you are living between two worlds—that is, you are physically here, but emotionally back home?

Do you participate or allow your children to participate in major holidays here in this country?

Do you think positively/negatively of your original culture?

Are you ashamed of your cultural background/accent/food/your relatives?

(For children) Do you feel ashamed/uncomfortable when your parents come to your school?

Do you feel that you do not want to have anything to do with this society?

Assess if the individual is identifying solely with his or her culture of origin.

Assess if the individual is depressed, angry, in transitional conflict, and so forth.

Assess if the individual has accepted the concept of biculturalism by asking about his or her interpersonal relations, cultural flexibility, respect for cultural differences, cultural transitional conflicts, and so forth.

Note if the individual is using only his or her homeland as a point of reference.

Request information on a child's school performance (academic, behavioral, and social) both in this country and in his or her country of origin. If you have to get the parents' permission to write the school in their native country, it is wise to do so.

Determine which stage of acculturation the individual is in (see Chapter 13 to further determine the stage).

Diagnosis:

Treatment Plan:

Determine whether the individual accepts counseling or is resistant. If he or she is resistant, try to explore the reason(s).

PART 2:
COMPARISON OF THE EDUCATION SYSTEMS

From primary through tertiary education, both the West Indian and the U.S. educational systems total 16 years of education (in the United States, kindergarten is not mandatory). The differences lie in the distribution of the years and the terminology used to describe various grades.

A question typically asked is which education system is better, the American or the West Indian. It is not a question of better or worse, but of differences. U.S. education is broader, so that by the end of elementary school the average child knows a little about many subjects, from computers and social studies to music and dance. In the West Indies, education at the elementary level is narrower but deeper, focusing mainly on mathematics and reading. U.S. education encourages discussion and more independent work at an earlier age. U.S. education is more visual, while West Indian education is more auditory. Examinations in the West Indies tend to be essays, while U.S. exams tend to be multiple-choice.

In the West Indies, after completing Form 5, the student has to take the Caribbean Examination Council (CXC) or the General Certificate Examination (GCE) in order to obtain a high school certificate (diploma). The student needs to pass at least five subjects (math and English must be passed) in order to be eligible for advanced education. The certificate indicates the student's level of performance in all the subjects taken. For the CXC, the grades range from 1 through 5, with 1, 2, and 3 acceptable for advanced education and employment. For the GCE, the grades are ranked A, B, C, D, and E, with A, B, and C the accepted levels for advanced education and employment. Students who do not reach the acceptable levels can retake the examination, which is usually given in January or June. When migrating to the United States, children should bring their high school transcripts, so that school administrators can assess their competence and the subject areas they studied.

In both the United States and the West Indies, a bachelor's degree is obtained upon completion of college or university.

Grade Equivalents

Age	United States	Most West Indian countries and U.S. Virgin Islands	St. Kitts/Nevis Jamaica
5	Kindergarten	ABC/1st year	Kindergarten
6	Grade 1	2nd year	Grade 1
7	Grade 2	Standard 1	Grade 2
8	Grade 3	Standard 2	Grade 3
9	Grade 4	Standard 3	Grade 4
10	Grade 5 Middle school begins in some areas	Standard 4	Grade 5
11	Grade 6 Junior high begins in some areas	Standard 5 High school begins	Grade 6 Junior high begins
12	Grade 7	Form 1	Form 1
13	Grade 8 High school begins for those attending middle school	Form 2	Form 2
14	Grade 9 High school begins for those attending junior high	Form 3	Form 3
15	Grade 10	Form 4	Form 4
16	Grade 11	Form 5	Form 5
17	Grade 12	Lower 6	Lower 6
18	1st year at college	Upper 6	Upper 6
19	2nd year at college	1st year at university	1st year at university
20	3rd year at college	2nd year at university	2nd year at university
21	4th year at college	3rd year at university	3rd year at university

Teachers in the United States ought to be aware of the following, based on a series of math textbooks for elementary schools—the *New Capital Arithmetic for the Caribbean* (Pierre, 1986)—and the Ministry of Education school syllabus:

By the end of Standard 1, students should be able to perform three-digit addition and subtraction, multiplication by up to 6, and division by up to 6. They should also know shapes and sizes, be able to tell time, and know currency units.

By the end of Standard 2, students should be able to add and subtract years and months, do multiplication by up to 12, multiply currency units, understand simple fractions and basic square measurements, and know the metric system.

By the end of Standard 3, students should know decimals, proper and improper fractions, mixed numbers, lowest common principles, and average.

By the end of Standard 4, students should understand weights, graphs, percentages, profits and loss, vulgar (common) fractions, shaping in proportion, and series.

By the end of Standard 5, students should know more difficult graphs, weights, approximation, prime factors and square roots, highest common factors, and lowest common factors.

At all grade levels children should be able to read phonetically, spell, know the parts of speech, and comprehend what they read. The level of difficulty depends on their grade.

Teachers should ask parents if their child has passed the common entrance exam (high school exam) and what school the child attended in the native country.

Parents ought to be careful that their children are not demoted upon entry into the U.S. school system. If a child is put back a grade, parents should ascertain the reason. For instance, they can ask if a test was given to the child to determine his or her grade placement.

Immigrant Self-Concept Scale*

AGES 11 AND OLDER

Participants must either have migrated from the West Indies to the United States, Canada, or Britain, or have parents who are immigrants from the West Indies.

Country of residence: United States   Canada   Britain

Were you born in this country?   Yes   No

If you answered "no" to the question above, what country in the West Indies are you from originally?

If you answered "yes" to the question above, what country or countries are your parents from originally?

Country of mother: Country of father:

Name (first name only):

Age: Grade/class (for children):

(For children) Father's occupation:
(For children) Mother's occupation:

(For adults) If you are employed, your occupation:
(For adults) If you are married, your spouse's occupation:

Gender: Male   Female

---

*Copyright © 1991 by Dr. Sharon-Ann Gopaul-McNicol.

Race: Black   White   Hispanic   Other

Socioeconomic status: Upper   Middle   Lower

(For children) Gender of your teacher: Male   Female

(For children) Race of your teacher: Black   White   Hispanic   Other

Below are statements about how you may or may not feel about yourself as an immigrant in the United States, Canada, or Britain. For each statement, please fill in the number that best shows how much you agree or disagree.

1 = Strongly disagree   2 = Disagree
3 = Neither agree or disagree   4 = Agree
5 = Strongly agree (a lot)

1. I think immigrants are lazy.

2. If I had one wish, I would wish that I was not an immigrant.

3. I do not like my West Indian accent.

4. I think immigrants are nice.

5. I think most immigrants are stupid.

6. I do not like being an immigrant.

7. I am proud to be an immigrant.

8. I think an immigrant person can succeed at anything he or she wants.

9. Immigrant people are just as honest as other people.

10. What I want more than anything is not to be an immigrant.

11. I do not like socializing with other immigrants.

12. Immigrant students can pass all their subjects in school if they study hard.

13. Most immigrants do bad things.

14. If I were in trouble, I would prefer a lawyer who is not an immigrant to defend me.

15. Being an immigrant does not keep me from being the best that I can be.

16. I feel that if I was not an immigrant, people would like me more.

17. No matter how much I try, I will fail because I am an immigrant.

18. Immigrants are just as intelligent as other people.

19. Because I am an immigrant I do not expect to have a good future.

20. All people are equal, regardless of their culture.

21. Immigrant teachers are just as good as teachers who are not immigrants.

22. If I were sick, I would prefer a doctor who is not an immigrant.

GRADES 1–4/AGES 6–10

Participants must either have migrated from the West Indies to the United States, Canada, or Britain, or have parents who are immigrants from the West Indies.

Country of residence: United States   Canada   Britain

Were you born in this country?   Yes   No

If you answered "no" to the question above, what country in the West Indies are you from originally?

If you answered "yes" to the question above, what country or countries are your parents from originally?

Country of mother: Country of father:

Name (first name only):

Age: Grade/class:

Gender: Male   Female

Race: Black   White   Hispanic   Other

Father's occupation: Mother's occupation:

Socioeconomic status: Upper   Middle   Lower

Gender of your teacher: Male   Female

Race of your teacher: Black   White   Hispanic   Other

Below are statements about how you may or may not feel about yourself as an immigrant in the United States, Canada, or Britain. For each statement, please tell me the degree to which you agree or disagree:

1 = Strongly disagree   2 = Disagree
3 = Neither agree or disagree   4 = Agree
5 = Strongly agree (a lot)

1. I think immigrants are lazy.

2. If I had one wish, I would wish that I was not an immigrant.

3. I do not like my West Indian accent.

4. I think immigrants are nice.

5. I think most immigrants are stupid.

6. I do not like being an immigrant.

7. I am proud to be an immigrant.

8. I think an immigrant person can succeed at anything he or she wants.

9. Immigrant people are just as honest as other people.

10. What I want more than anything is not to be an immigrant.

11. I do not like playing with other immigrant children.

12. Immigrant students can pass all their subjects in school if they study hard.

13. Most immigrants do bad things.

14. If I hurt myself, I would prefer that my parents took me to a doctor who is an immigrant.

15. The worst thing about me is that I am an immigrant.

16. I would really be happy if I was not an immigrant.

17. I feel that if I was not an immigrant, people would like me more.

18. The only thing that immigrants can do well is play sports.

19. I feel people will not accept me because I am an immigrant.

20. No matter how much I try, I will fail because I am an immigrant.

Immigrant Attitude Survey*

AGES 11 AND OLDER

Participants must either have migrated from the West Indies to the United States, Canada, or Britain, or have parents who are immigrants from the West Indies.

Country of residence: United States   Canada   Britain

Were you born in this country?   Yes   No

If you answered "no" to the question above, what country in the West Indies are you from originally?

If you answered "yes" to the question above, what country or countries are your parents from originally?

Country of mother: Country of father:

Name (first name only):

Age: Grade/class (for children):

(For children) Father's occupation:
(For children) Mother's occupation:

(For adults) If you are employed, your occupation:
(For adults) If you are married, your spouse's occupation:

Gender: Male   Female

---

*Copyright © 1991 by Dr. Sharon-Ann Gopaul-McNicol.

Race: Black   White   Hispanic   Other

Socioeconomic status: Upper   Middle   Lower

(For children) Gender of your teacher: Male   Female
(For children) Race of your teacher: Black   White   Hispanic   Other

Below are statements about how you may or may not feel about your cultural value system. Please put "True" or "False" next to the following statements. If you so desire, you can elaborate on any of them.

1 = True   2 = False

1. My parent(s)/I came to this country for a better life.

2. After I came here, I found it difficult to reunite with my family.

3. Black people are not as smart as white people.

4. If I had a choice, I would prefer to be white.

5. There are no racial problems in the West Indies.

6. The main problem in the West Indies is one of class.

7. A man should be considered the head of the home.

8. Women should stay at home and raise their children.

9. There are problems in marriages today because women have gone out in the workforce.

10. No matter what, couples should not get divorced.

11. Men are better able to handle money.

12. Men should be the main source of financial support in the home.

13. Abortion should not be legal.

14. Under certain circumstances, it is OK to have an abortion.

15. No matter what, men should support their children.

16. Women should be more responsible than men for disciplining children.

17. Men should be more responsible than women for disciplining children.

18. The older the child, the more responsibility he or she should have.

19. Younger children must listen to their older brothers and sisters.

20. Parents should be allowed to discipline their kids in any way they deem appropriate.

21. Spanking a child is not child abuse.

22. It should not make people uncomfortable to hug and kiss each other in the presence of others.

23. There is nothing inappropriate about a brother and sister sleeping in the same bed.

24. There is nothing wrong about children sleeping in the same bed as their parents.

25. There is nothing wrong with parents and children sleeping in the same room.

26. Children should not be allowed to leave home until they are ready to get married.

27. At what age do you think a person should leave home to live on his or her own? (Please put an age.)

28. Children should take care of their parents even after they leave home.

29. Teenage girls who become pregnant should leave school.

30. Teenage boys who are fathers should not stay in school.

31. Homosexuality is wrong.

32. Mental illness is something to be ashamed of.

33. As a child, it is not mature to cry if you are in pain.

34. As an adult, it is not mature to let others know that you are in pain.

35. It is wrong to discuss your family business (secrets) outside of your family.

36. Sex before marriage is wrong.

37. Growing up in the West Indies, I learned a lot about my country.

38. Growing up in the West Indies, I learned a lot about other islands in the West Indies.

39. The education in the country where I live now is better than the education in the West Indies.

40. When the British people were ruling the West Indies, the countries were better off.

41. It is better to work for the government than to take the risk of having your own business.

42. It is important to have a high school diploma.

43. It is important to get a college degree.

44. In the West Indies, a person can be anything he or she wants to be.

45. Success is obtaining a good job.

46. Success is getting a good education.

47. Rastafarian culture should not be respected.

48. The West Indian dialect is a respectable way of communicating in any setting.

49. The West Indian dialect should not be spoken in school.

50. If you have problems, it is better to talk to a priest than a counselor.

51. People who are said to be mentally ill are really possessed by evil spirits.

52. Arriving late for an appointment is not a big deal.

53. West Indians in this country are more ambitious than blacks who are from this country.

54. If a person can take care of himself or herself, such as cook and clean a house, he or she is not retarded.

A p p e n d i x   V

West Indian Attitude Survey*

AGES 11 AND OLDER

Participants must be West Indian citizens or have parents who are citizens of the West Indies.

Country of residence:

Were you born in this country?   Yes   No

If you answered "no" to the question above, what country in the West Indies are you from originally?

Name (first name only):

Age: Your class (for children):

(For children) Father's occupation:
(For children) Mother's occupation:

(For adults) If you are employed, your occupation:
(For adults) If you are married, your spouse's occupation:

Gender: Male   Female

Race: Black   White   Hispanic   Other

Socioeconomic status: Upper   Middle   Lower

(For children) Gender of your teacher: Male   Female

(For children) Race of your teacher: Black   White   Hispanic   Other

---

Below are statements about how you may or may not feel about your cultural value system. Please put "True" or "False" next to the following statements. If you so desire, you can elaborate on any of them.

1 = True   2 = False

1. There are no racial problems in the West Indies.

2. The main problem in the West Indies is one of class.

3. Black people are not as smart as white people.

4. If I had a choice, I would prefer to be white.

5. A man should be considered the head of the home.

6. Women should stay at home and raise their children.

7. There are problems in marriages today because women have gone out in the workforce.

8. No matter what, couples should not get divorced.

9. Men are better able to handle money.

10. Men should be the main source of financial support in the home.

11. Abortion should not be legal.

12. Under certain circumstances, it is OK to have an abortion.

13. No matter what, men should support their children.

14. Women should be more responsible than men for disciplining children.

15. Men should be more responsible than women for disciplining children.

16. The older the child, the more responsibility he or she should have.

17. Younger children must listen to their older brothers and sisters.

18. Parents should be allowed to discipline their kids in any way they deem appropriate.

19. Spanking a child is not child abuse.

20. It should not make people uncomfortable to hug and kiss each other in the presence of others.

21. There is nothing inappropriate about a brother and sister sleeping in the same bed.

22. There is nothing wrong about children sleeping in the same bed as their parents.

23. There is nothing wrong with parents and children sleeping in the same room.

24. Children should not be allowed to leave home until they are ready to get married.

25. At what age do you think a person should leave home to live on his or her own? (Please put an age.)

26. Children should take care of their parents even after they leave home.

27. Teenage girls who become pregnant should leave school.

28. Teenage boys who are fathers should not stay in school.

29. Homosexuality is wrong.

30. Mental illness is something to be ashamed of.

31. As a child, it is not mature to cry if you are in pain.

32. As an adult, it is not mature to let others know that you are in pain.

33. It is wrong to discuss your family business (secrets) outside of your family.

34. Sex before marriage is wrong.

35. Growing up in the West Indies, I learned a lot about my country.

36. Growing up in the West Indies, I learned a lot about other islands in the West Indies.

37. The education in Britain is better than the education in the West Indies.

38. When the British people were ruling the West Indies, the countries were better off.

39. It is better to work for the government than to take the risk of having your own business.

40. It is important to have a high school education.

41. It is important to go to university and obtain a bachelor's degree.

42. In the West Indies, a person can be anything he or she wants to be.

43. Success is obtaining a good job.

44. Success is getting a good education.

45. Rastafarian culture should not be respected.

46. The West Indian dialect is a respectable way of communicating in any setting.

47. The West Indian dialect should not be spoken in school.

48. If you have problems, it is better to talk to a priest than a counselor.

49. People who are said to be mentally ill are really possessed by evil spirits.

50. It is OK to arrive late for an appointment.

51. White people who live in this country are more ambitious than black people who are from this country.

52. If a person can take care of himself or herself, such as cook and clean a house, he or she is not retarded.

West Indian Community Services

Below are some recommended West Indian agencies in the New York City area that provide educational, social, economic, political, legal, or psychological services to families.

1. Caribbean Research Center, Medgar Evers College, City University of New York. Address—1150 Carroll St. Brooklyn, NY 11225. 718-270-6422. This is an academic and training institution set up to address the needs of the Caribbean-American population of New York State.

2. Caribbean Women's Health Association and Immigration Service Center. Address—2725 Church Ave. Brooklyn, NY 11226. 718-826-CWHA. This is a nonprofit organization whose mission is to inform, educate, and mobilize the public on crucial health-related issues affecting the Caribbean-American community. It also provides counseling and support services to assist immigrants in adjusting their status and becoming citizens.

3. Caribbean Chamber of Commerce and Industry. Address—26 Brooklyn Navy Yard, Brooklyn, NY 11226. 718-834-4544. This is a nonprofit group promoting economic development among Caribbean-American- and other minority-owned businesses. It also provides information and services necessary to fully develop the economic potential of minority entrepreneurs in the United States and the Caribbean nations.

4. Multicultural Educational and Psychological Services, P.C. Address—148 Greenwich St. Suite 103, Hempstead, NY 11550. 516-565-4015. This agency (which has offices in Long Island and Brooklyn) provides diagnostic, psychotherapeutic, and educational services to adults and children who are experiencing educational and adjustment difficulties. Most staff members are of West Indian background and are licensed psychologists in New York State.

5. Unique Christian Academy. Address—2222 Church St., Brooklyn, NY 11226. 718-856-0009. This is a school that educates children from prekindergarten through Grade 12; it is staffed by West Indian teachers.

6. Center for Immigrant Rights. 212-505-6890. This is the center for immigration matters, such as obtaining an attorney. The address is 48 St. Marks Place, New York, New York 10003.

References

Anderson, W., & Grant, R. (1987). *The new newcomers*. Toronto: Canadian Scholars Press.

Ambursley, F., & Cohen, R. (1983). *Crises in the Caribbean*. New York: Monthly Review Press.

American Psychiatric Association. (1987). *Diagnostic and statistical manual of mental disorders* (3rd ed., rev.). Washington, DC: Author.

Aponte, H. (1976). The family–school interview: An ecostructural approach. *Family Process, 15*(3), 303–311.

Aponte, H., & Van Deusen, J. (1981). Structural family therapy. In A. Gurman & D. Kniskern (Eds.), *Handbook of family therapy*. New York: Brunner/Mazer.

Armour-Thomas, E. (in press). Assessment in the service of thinking and learning for low achieving students. *High School Journal*.

Arredondo-Down, P. (1981). Personal loss and grief as a result of migration. *Personnel and Guidance Journal, 58*, 376–378.

Asby, D. (1975). Empathy: Let's get the hell on with it. *The Counseling Psychologist, 5*(2), 10–15.

Auerswald, E. (1968). Interdisciplinary versus ecological approach. *Family Process, 7*, 204.

Bandura, A. (1969). *Principles of behavior modification*. New York: Holt, Rinehart & Winston.

Baratz, S., & Baratz, J. (1970). Early childhood intervention: The social science base of institutional racism. *Harvard Educational Review, 40*, 29–50.

Bereton, B. (1985). *Social life in the Caribbean: 1838–1938*. London: Heinemann Kingston.

Bernal, M. (1991, October). Jamaica today. *American Visions*, pp. 2–6.

Berry, J. W., Kim, U., Minde, T., & Mok, D. (1987). Comparative studies of acculturative stress. *International Migration Review, 21*(3), 491–511.

Bowen, M. (1978). *Family therapy in clinical practice*. New York: Aronson.

Boyd-Franklin, N. (1989). *Black families in therapy*. New York: Guilford Press.

Brice, J. (1982). West Indian families. In M. McGoldrick, J. K. Pearce, & J. Giordano (Eds.), *Ethnicity and family therapy*. New York: Guilford Press.

Bronfenbrenner, U. (1977). Towards an experimental ecology of human development. *American Psychologist, 45*, 513–530.

Burke, J., & Tompkins, D. (1991, October). Reggae: Powerful journey. *American Visions*, pp. 10–11.

Charles, E. (1991). Effecting a regional plan for progress. *Caribbean Affairs, 4*(2), 25–30.

Christiansen, J., Thornley-Brown, A., & Robinson, J. (1984). *West Indians in Toronto*. Toronto: Family Service Association of Metropolitan Toronto.

Clark, K. B., & Clark, M. P. (1947). *Racial identification and preferences in Negro children*. New York: Holt.

Clarke, D. (1991). *The impact of foreign born inmates on the New York State Department of Correctional Services*. Albany: New York State Division of Program Planning, Research and Education.

Clarke, V., & Bolarinde, O. (1989). *Adjustment of Caribbean Immigrants in New York: Social and economic dimension*. New York: Caribbean Research Center.

Coelho, E. (1976). West Indian students in the secondary schools. *Tesl Talk, 7*(4), 37–46.

Coelho, E. (1991). *Caribbean students in Canadian schools*. Toronto: Pippin.

Cohen, Y. A. (1956). Structure and function: Family organization and socialization in a Jamaican community. *American Anthropologist, 58*, 664–680.

Craig, D. (1966). Teaching English to Jamaican Creole speakers: A model of a multi-dialect situation. *Language Learning, 16*(1–2), 49–61.

Cummings, J. (1984). *Bilingualism and special education: Issues in assessment and pedagogy*. San Diego: College Hill Press.

Daniel, E. (1952). *West Indian histories* (Vols. 1–3). London: Thomas Nelson & Sons.

De Albuquerque, K. (1979). The future of the Rastafarian movement. *Caribbean Review, 8*(4), 22.

DeFour, D. (1991). Issues in mentoring ethnic minority students. *Focus, 5*(1), 1–2.

Dillard, J. M. (1983). *Multicultural counseling*. Chicago: Nelson Hall.

Domokos-Cheng Ham, M. A. (1989a). Empathetic understanding: A skill for joining with immigrant families. *Journal of Strategic and Systemic Therapies, 8*(2), 36–40.

Domokos-Cheng Ham, M. A. (1989b). Family therapy with immigrant families: Constructuring a bridge between different world views. *Journal of Strategic and Systemic Therapies, 8*, 1–13.

Dumas, J. (1989). *Current demographic analysis of Caribbean immigrants in Canada*. Ottawa: Canadian Government Publishing Center.

Dunn, R., & Dunn, K. (1978). *Teaching students through their individual learning styles: A practical approach*. Reston, VA: Reston.

Dunn, R., Gemake, J., Jalali, F., & Zenhausern, R. (1990, April). Cross cultural differences of elementary age students from four ethnic backgrounds. *Journal of Multicultural Counseling and Development*, p. 18.

Edwards, V. K. (1979). *The West Indian student in British schools*. London: Routledge & Kegan Paul.

Edwards, W. F. (1983). Code selection and shifting in Guyana. *Language in Society, 12*(3), 290–297.

Elliot-Lewis, M. (1989). Responses to problems experienced by immigrant children. In V. Clarke & B. Obede (Eds.), *Adjustment of Caribbean immigrants in New York: Educational dimensions*. New York: Caribbean Research Center.

Ellis, A. (1974). *Humanistic psychotherapy: The rational emotive approach*. New York: McGraw-Hill.

Elliston, I. (1985). Counseling West Indian immigrants: Issues and answers. In R. Samuda & A. Wolfgang (Eds.), *Intercultural counseling and assessment: Global perspective*. Lewiston, NY: Hogrefe.

Erikson, E. (1980). *Identity and the life cycle*. New York: Norton.

Esquivel, G. (1985). *Best practices in the assessment of limited English proficient and bilingual children*. New York: Bilingual School Psychology Program, Fordham University.

Fabrega, H. (1969). Social psychiatric aspects of acculturation and migration. *Comprehensive Psychiatry, 10*(4), 314–326.

Falicov, C. (1988). Learning to think culturally in family therapy training. In H. Liddle, D. Breunlin, & R. C. Schwartz (Eds.), *Handbook of family therapy training and supervision*. New York: Guilford Press.

Figueroa, A. F., Sandoval, J., & Merino, B. (1984). School psychology and limited English proficient children: New competencies. *Journal of School Psychology, 22*, 133–143.

Friedman, E. (1982). The myth of Shiska. In M. McGoldrick, J. K. Pearce, & J. Giordano (Eds.), *Ethnicity and family therapy*. New York: Guilford Press.

Gibson, A. (1985). *A light in the dark tunnel*. London: Caribbean House.

Gibson, A. (1986). *The unequal struggle*. London: Caribbean House.

Giles, R. (1977). *The West Indian experience in British schools*. London: Heinemann.

Gladstein, G. (1983). Understanding empathy: Integrating counseling, developmental and social psychology perspective. *Journal of Counseling Psychology, 30*(4), 467–482.

Goodstein, C. (1990). America's cities: The new immigrants in the schools. *Crisis, 98*(5), 17–29.

Gopaul-McNicol, S. (1986). *The effects of modeling, reinforcement and color meaning word association of black preschool children and white preschool children in New York and Trinidad*. Unpublished doctoral dissertation, Hofstra University.

Gopaul-McNicol, S. (1988). Racial identification and racial preference of black preschool children in New York and Trinidad. *Journal of Black Psychology, 14*(2), 65–68.

Gopaul-McNicol, S. (1990, August). *The question of learning disability—Mental retardation or educational deprivation?* Paper presented at the annual meeting of the American Psychological Association, Boston.

Gopaul-McNicol, S., & Beckles, N. (1992). *The use of the Bender–Gestalt Visual–Motor Test with West Indian children.* Unpublished manuscript.

Gopaul-McNicol, S., & Shapiro, E. (1992). Understanding and meeting the psychological and educational needs of African American and Spanish speaking students. *School Psychology Review, 21*(4), 529–599.

Gopaul-McNicol, S., Thomas, T., & Irish, G. (1991). *A handbook for immigrants: Some basic educational and social issues in the United States of America.* New York: Caribbean Research Center.

Gordon, G. (1980). Bias and alternatives in psychological testing. *Journal of Negro Education, 49*(3), 350–360.

Gordon, H. (1960). *Report on the Rastafarian movement in Kingston, Jamaica.* Kingston, Jamaica: University of the West Indies.

Hartman, A. (1978). Diagrammatic assessment of family relationships. *Social Casework, 59*, 465–476.

Hartman, A., & Laird, J. (1983). *Family centered social work practice.* New York: Free Press.

Helms, J. (1985). Cultural identity in the treatment process. In P. Pedersen (Ed.), *Handbook of cross cultural counseling and therapy.* Westport, CT: Greenwood Press.

Hendriques, F. (1953). *Family and color in Jamaica.* London: Eyre & Spottiswoode.

Henry, F. (1982). A note on Caribbean migration to Canada. *Caribbean Review, 11*(1), 38.

Henry, F., & Wilson, P. (1975). Status of women in Caribbean societies: An overview of their social, economic and sexual roles. *Social and Economic Studies, 24*, 165–198.

Holman, A. (1983). *Family assessment: Tools for understanding and intervention.* Beverly Hills, CA: Sage.

Hunt, L. (1967). *Immigrants and the youth service.* London: Her Majesty's Stationery Office.

Jacobson, E. (1938). *Progressive relaxation.* Chicago: University of Chicago Press.

James, C. (1990). *Making it.* Oakville, Ontario: Mosaic Press.

James, S. (1978). When your patient is black West Indian. *American Journal of Nursing, 1978*, 1908–1909.

Justus, J. (1983). West Indians in Los Angeles: Community and identity. In R. Bryce-Laporte (Ed.), *Caribbean immigration into the United States.* Washington, DC: Smithsonian Institution.

Kerr, M. (1952). *Personality and conflict in Jamaica.* Liverpool, England: University Press.

Lamur, H., & Speckmann, J. (1975). *Adaptation of the migrants from the*

Caribbean in the European metropolis. Paper presented at the 34th annual conference of the American Association of Applied Anthropology, Amsterdam, The Netherlands.

Lazarus, A. A. (1976). *Multimodal behavior therapy*. New York: Springer.

Leary, P., & De Albuquerque, K. (1989). The other side of paradise: Race and class in the 1986 Virgin Islands elections. *Caribbean Affairs, 2*(1), 51–64.

Lefley, H. P. (1979). Prevalence of potential falling-out cases among Black, Latin and non-white populations of the city of Miami. *Social Science and Medicine, 13*(B), 113–128.

Leininger, M. (1973). Withcraft practices and psychocultural therapy with urban and United States families. *Human Organizations, 32*(1), 73–83.

Lewis, G. (1983). *Ten years of CARICOM*. Paper presented at a seminar sponsored by the Inter-American Development Bank, Washington, DC.

London, C. (1978). Sensitizing New York City teachers to the Caribbean student. In H. La Fontaine (Ed.), *Perspectives in bilingual education*. Garden City, NY: Avery.

London, C. (1980). *Teaching and learning with Caribbean students*. New York. (ERIC Document Reproduction Service No. ED 196 977).

London, C. (1983). Crucibles of Caribbean conditions: Factors for understanding for teaching and learning with Caribbean students in American educational settings. *Journal of Caribbean Studies, 2*(2–3), 182–188.

London, C. (1984, February–March). Caribbean turning point through education. *NOMMP: The Africana Studies and Research Center Newsletter*, pp. 1–2.

London, C. (1987). Ethnic composition of New York City schools. In A. Carrasquillo & E. Sandis (Eds.), *Schooling, job opportunities and ethnic mobility among Caribbean youth in the United States*. New York: The Equitable.

London, C. (1988). Educational theorizing in an emancipatory context. A case for Caribbean curriculum. *Journal of Caribbean Studies, 6*(2), 163–178.

London, C. (1989). *Through Caribbean eyes*. Chesapeake, VA: ECA Associates.

London, C. (1990). Educating young new immigrants: How can the United States cope? *International Journal of Adolescence and Youth, 2*, 81–100.

Mabey, C. (1981). Black British literacy. *Education Research, 23*(2), 83–95.

Mabey, C. (1986). Black pupils' achievement in inner city London. *Education Research, 28*(3), 163–173.

Marshall, D. (1982). The history of Caribbean migration: The case of the West Indies. *Caribbean Review, 11*(1), 6–11.

McGoldrick, M., Pearce, J. K., & Giordano, J. (Eds.). (1982). *Ethnicity and family therapy*. New York: Guilford Press.

McKenzie, M. (1986). Ethnographic findings on West Indian American clients. *Journal of Counseling Psychology, 65*, 40–44.

McNerney, M. (1979). The Trinidadian Creole speaker: Performance, awareness and attitude. *Tesl Talk, 10*(1–2).

McNerney, M. (1980). Teaching English to West Indian students: Developing a comprehensive yet differentiating approach. *Tesl Talk*, *11*(1), 26–32.

McNicol, M. (1991). *Helping children adjust to a new culture: A child's perspective.* New York: Multicultural Educational and Psychological Services.

Meichenbaum, D. H. (1977). *Cognitive-behavior modification.* New York: Plenum Press.

Mercer, J. R. (1973). *Labelling the mentally retarded.* Berkeley: University of California Press.

Miller, E. L. (1967). *A study of body image, its relationship to self-concept, anxiety and certain social and physical variables in a selected group of Jamaican adolescents.* Unpublished master's thesis, University of the West Indies, Kingston, Jamaica.

Minuchin, S. (1974). *Families and family therapy.* Cambridge, MA: Harvard University Press.

Minuchin, S., Montalvo, B., Guerney, B. G., Jr., Rosman, B. L., & Schumer, F. (1967). *Families of the slums.* New York: Basic Books.

Mollica, R. F., Wyshak, G., & Lowelle, J. (1987). The psychosocial impact of war trauma and torture on southeast Asian refugees. *American Journal of Psychiatry*, *144*(12), 1567–1572.

New York City Department of Planning, Office of Immigrant Affairs and Population Analysis Division. (1985). *Caribbean immigrants in New York City: A demographic summary.* Unpublished manuscript.

New York City Police Department. (1985). Rasta crime. *Caribbean Review*, *14*(1), 12.

Parry, J., Sherlock, P., & Maingot, A. (1987). *A short history of the West Indies* (4th ed.). London: Macmillan.

Pasternak, M. (1986). *Helping kids learn multicultural concepts: A handbook of strategies.* Champaign, IL: Research Press.

Payne, M. (1989). Use and abuse of corporal punishment: A Caribbean view. *Child Abuse and Neglect*, *13*, 389–401.

Pedersen, P. (Ed.). (1985). *Handbook of cross cultural counseling and therapy.* Westport, CT: Greenwood Press.

Philippe, J., & Romain, J.B. (1979). Indisposition in Haiti. *Social Science and Medicine*, *13*(B), 129–133.

Phillips, A. S. (1976). *Adolescence in Jamaica.* Kingston, Jamaica: Jamaica Publishing House.

Pierre, A. (1986). *New capital arithmetic for the Caribbean.* Kingston, Jamaica: Heinemann.

Plowden, L. (1967). *The Plowden report: Children and their primary schools.* London: Department of Education and Science and Her Majesty's Stationery Office.

Raspberry, W. (1991, May 14). Right strategies for wrong countries. *New York Daily News*, p. 35.

Regional Newspaper for the North Eastern Caribbean. (1991, September 16). Trinidad plans to fight deportation.

Rimer, S. (1991, September 16). Between two worlds: Dominicans in New York. *New York Times*, p. B6–L.

Roberts, P. (1988). *West Indians and their language*. London: Cambridge University Press.

Rodney, W. (1983). *The groundings with my brothers*. London: Bogle-L'Ouverture Publications.

Rogers, C. (1975a). What is Rasta? *Caribbean Review*, 7(1), pp. 1–12.

Rogers, C. (1975b). Empathetic: An unappreciated way of being. *The Counseling Psychologist*, 5(2), 2–10.

Ronstrom, A. (1989). Children in Central America: Victims of war. *Child Welfare League of America*, 58(2), 145–153.

Rosenthal, R., & Jacobson, L. (1968). *Pygmalion in the classroom*. New York: Holt, Rinehart & Winston.

Saakana, A. S., & Pearse, A. (1986). *Towards the decolonization of the British educational system*. London: Frontline Journal/Karnak House.

Samuda, R. (1975). From ethnocentrism to a multicultural perspective in educational testing. *Journal of Afro-American Issues*, 3(1), 4–17.

Scobie, E. (1972). *Black Britannia*. Chicago: Johnson.

Semaj, L. (1979). Inside Rasta: The future of a religious movement. *Caribbean Review*, 14(1), 8.

Sewell-Coker, B., Hamilton-Collins, J., & Fein, E. (1985, November). Social work practice with West Indian immigrants. *Social Casework: Journal of Contemporary Social Work*, pp. 563–568.

Short, G. (1985). Teacher expectation and West Indian underachievement. *Educational Research*, 27(2), 95–101.

Silvera, M. (1986). *Silenced*. Toronto: Williams Wallace.

Skinner, B. F. (1974). *About behaviorism*. New York: Knopf.

Solomon, P. (1992). *Black resistance in high school*. Albany: State University of New York Press.

Soutar-Hynes, M. (1976). West Indian realities in the intermediate grades: The emerging role of the ESD teacher. *Tesl Talk*, 7(4), 31–36.

Sowell, T. (1981). *Ethnic America*. New York: Basic Books.

Stewart, R. (1986). *The United States in the Caribbean*. Kingston, Jamaica: Heinemann.

Sue, S. (1981). *Counseling the culturally different*. New York: Wiley.

Sue, S., & Zane, N. (1987). The role of culture and cultural techniques in psychotherapy. *American Psychologist*, 55, 37–45.

Thomas, T. (1991, August). *Post traumatic stress disorder in children*. Paper presented at the annual meeting of the American Psychological Association, Boston.

Thomas, T., & Gopaul-McNicol, S. (1991). *An immigrant handbook on special education in the United States of America*. New York: Multicultural Educational and Psychological Services.

Thrasher, S., & Anderson, G. (1988, March). The West Indian family: Treatment challenges. *Social Casework: Journal of Contemporary Social Work*, pp. 171–176.

Triandis, H., & Brislin, R. (1984). Cross cultural psychology. *American Psychologist, 52*, 1006–1009.

Troike, R. (1968). Social dialects and language learning: Implications for TESOL. *TESOL Quarterly, 2*(3), 176–180.

Valere-Meredith, J. (1983). *Factors involved in the pidginization process of the English negative system.* Unpublished manuscript.

Valere-Meredith, J. (1985). *Problems in the methodology in the teaching of English as a second dialect.* Unpublished manuscript.

Valere-Meredith. J. (1989). *Teaching English as a second dialect for illiterate West Indians in Canada.* Unpublished manuscript.

Walker, J. (1984). *The West Indians in Canada.* Ottawa: Keystone.

Waters, A. M. (1984). *Race, class and political symbols.* New Brunswick, NJ: Transaction Books.

Weidman, H. (1979). Falling-out: A diagnostic and treatment problem viewed from a transcultural perspective. *Social Science and Medicine, 13*(B), 95–112.

Whitaker, C. (1986). The West Indian influence. *Ebony, 41*(7), 135–144.

Williams, E. (1967). *Capitalism and slavery.* London: Lowe & Brydone.

Williams, E. (1981). *Forge from the love of liberty.* Port of Spain, Trinidad: Longman Caribbean.

Williams, R. (1971). Abuses and misuses in testing black children. *Washington University Magazine, 41*(3), 34–37.

Williams, R. (1980). Scientific racism and IQ: The silent mugging of the black community. *Psychology Today, 7*(12), 32–41.

Wittkower, E. D. (1964). Spirit possession in Haitian voodoo ceremonies. *Acta Psychotherapeutica, 12*, 72–80.

Yekwai, D. (1988). *British racism: Miseducation and the Afrikan child.* London: Karnak House.

Young, L., & Bagley, C. (1979). *Identity, self-esteem and evaluation of color and ethnicity in young children in Jamaica and London.* Paper presented at the Third annual conference of the Society of Caribbean Studies, London.

Index